True Homœopathy

Dr. Samuel Hahnemann's
Original Homœopathic Medicine

NICOLA HENRIQUES

Ordering Information:
Visit www.createspace.com to order more copies

True Homœopathy/Nicola Henriques—1st ed.
ISBN: 978-0-9985192-0-3

DISCLAIMER

The purpose of this book is to educate. While every effort has been made to make it as complete and accurate as possible, the content should be used only as a general guide. Readers are advised to use their own judgement and consult their personal physicians regarding individual particular health problems and symptoms. The author and publisher shall have neither liability nor responsibility to any person or entity regarding any loss or damage caused, or alleged to have been caused, directly or indirectly, by information contained in this book.

Faithful to the end

Contents

Efficiency in homœopathy implies and involves native ability, acquired technical proficiency, and logical consistency in the application of its principles. The exercise of these qualifications requires honesty, courage, fidelity to a high ideal and a right point of view.

Dr. Stuart Close, *The Genius of Homœopathy*

Author's Preface

I have always been a critical thinker, someone who delves, challenges, interrogates and goes against the grain of popular opinion to find the truth.

I wrote this book to eliminate the shroud of baseless confusion and mystery that envelopes homœopathy, and help those interested in receiving and providing effective homœopathic treatment understand how to use homœopathic medicines to best advantage. I also want to raise public and practitioner awareness of the highest standard of homœopathic clinical excellence established by Dr. Samuel Hahnemann, the originator of homœopathy.

A man of science Hahnemann never intended for homœopathy to be mysterious. To provide clarity regarding every aspect of homœopathy, he published detailed explanations of its science, doctrine, laws of nature, processes, method and rules in various books and articles. After forty-seven years of clinical practice Hahnemann brought all the information together in the Sixth final revision of *The Organon of Medicine,* his treatise on health, disease and how to restore lasting health using homœopathy. In that document Hahnemann provides a clear definition of what homœopathy is, what it is not, what it can achieve and its limitations, and explains exactly how to practise homœopathy in the true sense of the word, and how homœopathic medicines are able to transform illness into health.

Furthermore, Hahnemann understood full well that for homœopathy to be accepted as a legitimate medical system in its own right, it must prove its effectiveness and to do that it must meet science's reasonable demand for consistency in methodology. For that reason and to ensure detractors and sceptics of homœopathy could not reproach us for not having a normal standard of clinical practice, Hahnemann practised, taught and promulgated a single doctrine of homœopathy, rooted in pure experiments, and a single method of practice based on certain fixed, plain, intelligible, fundamental principles which govern every aspect of homœopathic practice, and must be properly understood, rigorously adhered to and consistently applied to every individual case of disease.[1] Devoid of divergence and distortion, this principle based non routine form of prescribing homœopathic medicines is the only methodology that Hahnemann considered worthy of the honourable name "Homœopathy,"[2] and the standard of clinical excellence he fiercely asserted all true practitioners of homœopathy should always apply and their patients should always receive.

Hahnemann could not force prescribers of homœopathic medicines to read, understand and conscientiously follow his instructions, but he hoped that we would.

As homœopathy struggles to avoid abolition and build an evidence base proving its effectiveness, it is worth remembering Hahnemann invited all his critics to test the efficacy of homœopathy conscientiously, honestly and fairly without divergence, distortion, modification, prejudice or trickery. He knew the best way to do that was to apply his methodology *exactly*, and he provided this simple, refreshingly prescriptive formula and reason for doing so:

> Take one disease after another strictly according to the principles and directions given in *The Organon of Medicine*. Note down the case, especially in respect of all the discoverable symptoms, in so exact a manner that the founder of homœopathy himself shall be unable to find fault with the accuracy of the report … and administer pure and unmixed, the most appropriate homœopathic medicinal substance that can be discovered for the case of disease in question, in a dose as small as this doctrine directs, but, as is expressly insisted on, *taking care to remove all other kinds of medicinal influences from the patient*; and if it does not give relief, speedy, mild, and permanent relief, then by a publication of the duly attested history of the

[1] Dr. Samuel Hahnemann, *The Organon of Medicine*, Sixth edition, Author's Preface & §2

[2] Ibid., Author's Preface

treatment according to the principles of the homœopathic system strictly followed out, you will be able to give a public refutation of this doctrine which so seriously threatens the old darkness.

But I pray you to beware of playing false in the matter!—all roguery comes to light and leaves an indelible stigma behind it as a warning.

If then, following your conscientious example, every other equally conscientious and careful medical experimentalist meets with the same result … then homœopathy is as good as lost; it is all up with homœopathy if it does not show itself efficacious, remarkably efficacious.[3]

By presenting Dr. Samuel Hahnemann's original medical masterpiece: '*The Pure Homœopathic Healing Art*' in its pristine state, I want to uphold the honour and dignity of homœopathy and show you the majesty, elegance and logic of his incomparable homœopathic practice methodology. Most importantly, I will demonstrate how ineffectiveness and obstacles to recovery are created when the rules, processes, principles and controls Hahnemann put in place to underpin the functionality and durability of homœopathy, are unknown or misunderstood, ignored, altered, dismantled, abandoned and dismissed.

NICOLA HENRIQUES

The reader will note, the classical form of "homœopathy"—keeping the "œ" ligature—is used throughout the text, except where the "Americanized" word "homeopathy" or the European version "homoeopathy" is used in direct quotations or titles of publications. This book includes thoroughly revised and expanded material from previous works by the same author.

---

[3] Dr. S. Hahnemann, *Materia Medica Pura*

Introduction

Long before the current global catastrophe of drug resistant illness, German physician, Christian Friedrich Samuel Hahnemann (1755–1843), drew attention to the harmful side effects produced by prolonged overuse of large physiological doses of drugs by ordinary medical practitioners.

To address the problem, Dr. Hahnemann argued for a major rethink of Western medical practice. To lead the way he originated a completely new medical system based on the theory of vitalism: the theory that the origin and phenomena of life are dependent on a force or principle distinct from purely chemical or physical forces, and the therapeutic law of Nature: *Let likes be cured with likes*—the treatment of symptoms produced naturally during illness with the single smallest dose of a single medicinal substance which, when given to healthy people, produces the greatest number of symptoms similar to those experienced. Hahnemann named the new medical system Homœopathy derived from two Greek words *homoios* and *pathos*, meaning "similar" and "suffering."

There is much more to homœopathy than prescribing micro doses of medicines according to the principle of like cures like. Homœopathy is the epitome of personalised medical treatment. Just as detectives and forensic scientists at crime scenes painstakingly interview witnesses, look for clues and build profiles of possible perpetrators, pure homœopathic healing artists use inductive methods of research and deductive reasoning while eliciting each person's illness history, detecting characteristic individualised symptoms, then taking that morass of information analysing it and assembling the information in such a way that it creates a unique multidimensional "mug shot" portrait of each person's particular mental, emotional and physical suffering. Then the practitioner carefully searches the homœopathic equivalent of a 'mug-shot' database for the description of a single medicinal substance with a proven record of inducing the greatest number of symptoms similar to those experienced. After that, careful consideration is given to selection of the proper dose and intervals between doses that will induce gentle, rapid longlasting recovery.

Whether patients are humans or animals, each phase of homœopathic treatment demands intense collaboration between practitioner, and the patient or their guardian. For homœopathy to achieve its mission of rapid, gentle, continuous recovery, and sustainable health with minimal medicine, both must view the illness from their own vantage points and think very deeply about the state of suffering experienced or observed. The degree of intelligence applied by a practitioner profoundly affects the quality of information offered, gleaned and evaluated and the violent or gentle, continuous or intermittent, slow or rapid pace of recovery using homœopathic medicines.

Hahnemann's teaching style is not for the faint-hearted. He set a high bar for patient safety, practitioner technical proficiency and due diligence. He is the teacher who always demands the very best from all his students, who knows we have a lot to offer if only we would knuckle down and give it our best shot. We might hate him at the time, but later on we may realise he is the only teacher who will never give up on us, and will always be there when we need him most.

Mastery of homœopathy is inextricably linked to the practitioner's scholarship of Hahnemann's *The Organon of Medicine,* Sixth final edition,[4] the handbook, operating system manual and blueprint for homœopathy, where he clearly articulates and systematically sets down the fixed fundamental principles, laws, rules and processes derived from pure experiments, that form a coherent body of knowledge about homœopathy and its methodology. This is where Hahnemann cuts

---

[4] All quotes are from the 1921 unadulterated English translation by Dr. William Boericke

through to the core of the truth of homœopathy, where he clarifies what homœopathy is and what it is not, explains how homœopathic medicines work, as well as:

- How to uncover the medicinal qualities of substances
- How to prepare the medicines for the purpose of health restoration
- How to relate to patients
- How to examine patients
- How to document information
- How to properly select the most suitable homœopathic medicine and dosage
- How to select proper intervals between each dose
- How to evaluate patient responses to medicines
- The most common practitioner errors, how and why we make them and how to correct them quickly
- The obstacles to be surmounted or removed when treating illness.

In *The Organon of Medicine,* Hahnemann identifies the most common practitioner errors, explains how, when and why we are likely to make them and how to correct them quickly, as well as addressing other obstacles to be surmounted when treating illness. He exhorts practitioners to stop adapting homœopathy to fit the flawed view of health, disease and cure held by ordinary medical practitioners. The completeness of this work begs the following question: how is it so many prescribers openly admit they do not understand how homœopathic medicines work and, there are no rules governing the practice of homœopathy?

To acquire the knowledge about homœopathy contained in *The Organon of Medicine,* six distinct intellectual skills are required by teacher and student alike: critical thinking, the capacity to read, absorb, understand what has been read, and to retain it. Where those skills are absent in teachers, untaught and undeveloped in students, or not enough attention is paid to the different ways and time it takes for students to learn, students fail to fully understand the principle of homœopathy, the most important book on homœopathy is misperceived as boring and impenetrable, and so cast aside. Instead of deciding to stretch our mind, we begin the endless search for the gadget or guru that will allow us to understand homœopathy instantaneously, with complete clarity without any intellectual effort, and in so doing expose ourselves to the many false doctrines taught under the name homœopathy that exist.

As a student and a teacher I found it more useful to consider that since nature makes an enormous effort to ensure our survival, it might be wise to match that effort in order to protect patients lives, and that there is a striking similitude between the Herculean effort of concentration required to mine the depths of *The Organon of Medicine* and the Herculean effort required to mine the depths of each person's illness. This perspective provides insight into Hahnemann's objectives: to inculcate in students and practitioners a propensity for perseverance and effort, rigour, self-discipline, and inordinate intellectual acuity, so that we are suitably prepared for the exacting challenges ahead. Once hubris is replaced with humility and we begin to synchronise our view of cure and health with that of Hahnemann's, boredom is banished, confusion is replaced by clarity and studying *The Organon of Medicine* becomes an intellectually enriching experience. This is why expertly guided in depth study of *The Organon of Medicine* is an essential part of training to become a true practitioner of homœopathy.

This book will bring you to a deeper understanding of homœopathy and in that way increase the opportunity for patients to experience an enduring level of health restoration. You will learn how to hone the intellect into the precision tool required to homœopathically select the most suitable symptom-similar medicine, proper dose and correct intervals between doses for each individual and their illness. You will understand what happens after a homœopathic medicine is ingested and why, what action to take next and why, and how to identify, avoid or quickly correct mistakes. You will understand why simple illnesses may become extremely complicated and how they may be managed confidently. In Hahnemann's words, you will learn how to treat illness judiciously and rationally and what it takes to become a true practitioner of the healing art of homœopathy.[5]

---

[5] Dr. S. Hahnemann, *The Organon of Medicine*, §3

1

Easily Comprehensible Principles

To ensure each patient's experience of homœopathy is sweet and not sour, and the medical system of homœopathy achieves the highest ideal of cure: rapid, gentle and continuous restoration of health, or removal and annihilation of a disease in its whole extent, in the shortest, most reliable, and most harmless way,[6] Hahnemann required all practitioners to observe and apply the following fundamental principles to every case of disease:

1. The Vital Force of Nature
2. Inherent predispositions to illness
3. Susceptibility: action and reaction
4. Totality of characteristic individualising symptoms
5. Smallest dose: dilution and potentiation
6. Know the curative power of each individual medicine
7. Let likes be cured with likes—*Similia Similibus Curentur*
8. Proper dose: single substance, single dose
9. Natural direction of cure

These principles are the hallmarks of homœopathy. Each fixed principle is an integral inseparable part of the whole medical system of

---

[6] Dr. Samuel Hahnemann, *The Organon of Medicine*, Sixth edition, §2

homœopathy. To easily grasp their significance, think of them as the highest quality material used to construct, strengthen and support the edifice on which the science and art of homœopathy are built. Allow ignorance, omission, alteration or perversion of any of the fixed principles and the edifice crumbles into dust.

In totality these principles:

- Serve as the chain of reasoning that underpins the origination, structure and practice of homœopathy
- Have always been the same and will always remain the same
- Are the mainstays of homœopathy
- Are rules that govern best-practice homœopathy and provide a normal prescribing standard
- Provide medical science with consistency of methodology
- Correct flawed thinking about homœopathy
- Provide a benchmark against which to assess and compare divergent methodologies and identify false doctrines
- Guide practitioners through each phase of treatment ensuring avoidance of roundabout methods, speculation, guesswork, empiricism and routine use of drugs

To thoroughly understand the following information without being overwhelmed by it, pace yourself. You want your knowledge to grow gently, steadily and deeply. My advice is don't skim read. Take your time. Read each principle and ponder it for a while, when it makes sense to you, tackle the next one and so on. Gradually you will see how each principle dovetails with the next to form a solid framework for the homœopathic thought process. When they are understood and applied in their totality they allow practitioners to:

- Know the things that derange, alter health, and cause disease
- Know what is to be cured in each individual case of disease
- Know the curative powers of each medicine
- Know how to adapt natural substances for medicinal purposes
- Know how to select each medicine for each sick person
- Know how to select the appropriate dose and correct period for repeating each dose

- Know how to identify obstacles to recovery and develop strategies for their removal[7]

Effective practitioners of true homœopathy are able to sustain long periods of intense concentration and clarity of perspective during each phase of treatment; are able to view each individual's experience of disease as being unique, never ever seen by them before; know what the obstacles to recovery are in each case and how to remove them; are able to understand the evolution of each individual's illness in its whole extent—from the earliest signs of trouble through to the moment the patient seeks help, and up to and including restoration of continuous health.

The first four principles: *Vital Force of Nature; Inherent Predispositions to illness; Susceptibility: action and reaction; Totality of characteristic individualising symptoms of the illness,* show us how to conduct the most effective homœopathic patient examination so that we know exactly what needs to be understood about each patient and the unique nature of the illness to be treated, and we elicit the central disturbance. Their rigorous application provides practitioner knowledge of the following:

- Things that alter health and cause illness
- Things that indicate disease
- The individual's strength or weakness at a given moment

Let's explore each fundamental principle in detail.

Vital Force of Nature

Understanding the principle of vitalism Hahnemann recognised that an invisible, powerful, intangible force of nature distinct from purely chemical or physical forces, exists within every molecule and it is that operative power or energy which changes the state of matter within the living organism.

Present throughout the body, this vital force of nature instinctively preserves life; is the innate self-healing power each of us possesses and motivates us to achieve our full spiritual, mental, emotional and physical

---

[7] Dr. S. Hahnemann, *The Organon of Medicine,* Sixth edition, §1 to §4.

potential in life. It is often described as Qi or Prana and experienced as vitality, vital energy, high or low spirits. The natural direction of this vital force is always inwards outward. Absence of this vital force is observed in a corpse. In homœopathy, cure will be certain and rapid in proportion to the strength with which the vital force still prevails in the patient.[8]

The vital force is strongest when the progress of life is unimpeded. Without the need of medicine of any kind, this force naturally instinctively corrects minor imbalances and reduces susceptibility to illness. Even though we are exposed to a multitude of harmful influences every hour of every day, we withstand most of them. We will feel 'off' for a short while, then—still without medication—we rapidly bounce back, showing us nature is at work. Our vital force is fulfilling its mission to sustain and preserve life.

On the understanding that no medicine has been ingested, persisting discomfort in one or more regions of the body provides evidence of a disproportionate susceptibility to some extremely harmful influence(s). Left alone without help, the vital force is powerless to resist or efficiently restore balance. The appearance of each symptom experienced during a person's lifetime and the distinctive extremes of suffering in different regions of the body, indicates an unresolved continuously progressing single state of disharmony and dis-ease affecting the entire person. A single symptom no more represents the whole disease than a single foot represents the whole person. It is the totality of uncomfortable changes that constitutes a particular person's disease and it is the totality that must be treated.[9] The complete illness history spans the entire period of time—from the first moment the person feels unwell, the first time symptoms appeared, the oldest symptoms through to the most recent symptoms, the moment they start treatment and beyond. The length of time that symptoms have been experienced indicates how long the vital force has been struggling to restore balance and preserve life without help.

---

[8] Dr. Samuel Hahnemann, *The Organon of Medicine*, Sixth edition, Author's Preface

[9] Ibid §7

Homœopathy is designed to treat and remove symptoms of natural illness that occur when a particular set of conditions exists: there is an inherent predisposition to disease that has become extremely aggravated and, as it were, opened a window of disproportionate psychological and physical susceptibility to powerful harmful influences. In that moment of increased susceptibility, the vital force is overpowered by the harmful influence(s), and completely surrenders. The previous balance and integrity of our whole being is now weakened and damaged.[10] Life is threatened, the vital force panics. To rid itself of the harm, every orifice in the body is used as a vent: ears, eyes, nose, mouth, skin pores, rectum, etc. Fever is quelled by perspiration and increased secretion of urine. Lung inflammation is soothed by increased mucus, perspiration and often nosebleeds. Tonsil inflammation is reduced by increased salivation. Other venting tactics include enlargement of glands, coughing, vomiting, diarrhoea and bleeding from the anus, and skin eruptions. If none of that works, the vital force goes into damage limitation mode. Sometimes the harmful influence is contained within tumours, cysts, secondary growths, and stashed around the body to be dealt with when there is more energy.

In homœopathy, experience of symptoms is considered to be evidence that the natural curative process is definitely underway, but that the vital force has run out of steam. It has stalled, rather than not started at all and is now exhausted, crawling around on hands and knees, crying out for help to finish the job it started. The remaining energy must be conserved and nurtured. A fragile vital force must be gently strengthened and nudged into curative activity with the smallest medicinal dose—rather than being given a violent kick in the pants with the largest dose of ordinary or homœopathic medicines, which often completely overwhelms it for a second time. Least medicine is best medicine. The correctly selected homœopathic medicine is one that works in union with and boosts the remaining power of the vital force, enabling it to free itself from harm.

For the proper smallest dose of homœopathic medicine to be selected, practitioner knowledge of the unique state of each patient's

---

[10] Ibid §31 and Author's Preface to the Fourth edition, *The Organon of Medicine*

vital force at the time of presentation is essential. The dose must be just sufficient—no more, no less—to engage the vital force in repairing the damage it caused and thus transform illness into health.

Knowledge about the prevailing strength of the vital force is obtained through the location and intensity of each symptom experienced. When the vital force is disturbed, depending on its strength or weakness at a given moment, the centre and degree of the disturbance manifests itself in the spiritual, intellectual, emotional spheres or physical body. Where most of the suffering is in the interior of the body, it is understood that the strength of the vital force is severely reduced. It has insufficient strength to resist, protect the inner regions of the body from harm and push the central disturbance to the peripheral regions. Where most of the suffering occurs in the outer regions, the vital force is judged to be somewhat stronger. It has sufficient energy to keep the disorder in these outer regions but insufficient energy to completely expel the harm and restore health.

Put another way, viewing the individual from innermost to outermost regions the extreme innermost region is the energy at the core of our being, otherwise known as our invisible vital force, the mental faculties encompassing our will, intellect, desires longings, cravings, aversions and hatreds, fears dreads, etc. Closest to the innermost region is the brain and central nervous system. Moving progressively further and further away from the innermost regions, we next look at the vital organs, fluids, gases associated with the endocrine, reticuloendothelial, circulatory, lymphatic, respiratory, digestive, urinary, reproductive, skeletal, muscular and outer protective layers. Therefore, where the region(s) most affected by long-continued illness involve the innermost, the vital force is perceived to be weak and insufficient, lacking power to repel or push the harmful disturbance outwards to the furthest regions of the body. Where the region most affected is the protective, outer layer, the vital force is considered to be much stronger and capable of completing cure almost unassisted.

In homœopathy, every uncomfortable sensation or symptom experienced is the vital force shouting for help. They give us precise information about the location, nature, character, degree, depth and extent of the trouble. Each symptom described and gleaned during the patient examination process is evaluated for usefulness in the creation of a unique portrait of illness to identify the single symptom-similar medicine pertinent to each patient. Proper administration of the smallest dose of that medicine has the potential to remove the whole of that particular individual's suffering. Changes described by the patient after ingestion of the medicine are the practitioner's only useful guide to understanding the curative versus the non-curative response of the vital force to the remedy and dose.

A practitioner's failure to observe, or misinterpretation of, the distress signals of the vital force, and ignoring its significant role in maintaining health, causing and curing disease leads to avoidable mistakes and obstacles to recovery including:

- Ignorance about what is to be cured in disease
- Misunderstanding, or misjudgment of, the prevailing strength of the VF
- Imperfect remedy or dose selection
- The improper period for remedy dose repetition
- The failure to effect cure

Inherent predispositions to illness

The second fixed principle relates to causations and traits of illness. In homœopathy, there are three main causations: *exciting* (e.g. shock, trauma, epidemics, etc.), *maintaining* (e.g. work, domestic violence, war, iatrogenic disease, lack of love, food, heat, light, clean water or air, etc.) and *fundamental* inherent predispositions to illness or 'miasms'[11] infectious or noxious emanations.

Hahnemann originated homœopathy to achieve rapid, gentle, continuous or permanent restoration of health rather than temporary relief from symptoms. After practising for some years, he observed that even with the best homœopathic treatment, some individuals fell ill again after recovering. To understand why this happened, Hahnemann spent fifteen years investigating the nature of individual constitutions and diseases that have affected the human race throughout history. He

---

[11] 19th Century German word, from the Greek, miasma: defilement.

deduced that it was inherent, unceasing, fluctuating, latent or dormant harmful influences that predispose us to certain illnesses.

Passed from generation to generation, these inherent predispositions bond with the vital force and leave their indelible marks on our constitution. Murder is their mission. They often remain unrecognised for years, especially when we're young and flourishing, and enjoying a lifestyle that is beneficial to our soul, heart and body. We look and feel as if we're in perfect health. Later on, after some adverse or life-changing event, these dispositions re-emerge in a new disguise. In proportion to the degree they have weakened or disturbed the vital force, they develop rapidly and assume a more serious character, especially when the vital force has been medically mismanaged.[12] Prolonged medical treatment and violent, strong medicines sap the patient's vitality to an unmerciful extent, rendering the vital force incapable of responding to homœopathic medicine and the patient incurable.[13]

Slumbering inherent predispositions to illness may also be awakened by improper administration of very high doses of incorrectly chosen homœopathic medicines repeated too frequently and without their effects being properly monitored.

A proficient homœopathic patient examination includes a review of the family medical history. This tracks the path of destruction wrought by the predispositions to the moment they first got a grip on the patient. The symptom history reveals the traces, identity of each predisposition and determines which one dominates the case at that specific time. It also reveals whether its influence is latent, slowed, suspended or active. In homœopathic practice, the more complicated an illness is, the more likely it is that the illness is caused by the harmful influence of multiple inherent predispositions. Effective treatment involves calming the activity of the predispositions and, where possible, annihilating them—gently teasing apart these threads and loosening a knot. Multiple predispositions produce more threads and tighter knots.

---

[12] Dr. S. Hahnemann, *The Organon of Medicine* Sixth revised edition, §78 and footnote 76

[13] Ibid, §74

Hahnemann understood that three inherent predispositions (miasms) are responsible for all chronic illnesses.[14] They are named 'Sycosis', from the Greek word sycon for 'fig' or 'figwart', because its sequelae resemble overgrowth of tissue, figwart-like, symptoms. The second is called 'Syphilis', due to its manifestation of destructive, ulcerating tendencies and symptoms, which closely resemble those produced in the venereal disease. The third predisposition is named 'Psora' the Latin, Greek word for itch, and is responsible for itching skin conditions and prolonged, recurring illnesses.

In terms of which one is most problematic, according to Hahnemann:

> At least seven-eighths of all chronic maladies spring from Psora as their only source, while the remaining eighth spring from Syphilis and Sycosis or from a complication of two of these three miasmatic chronic diseases, or (which is rare) from a complication of all three of them.[15]

If we think of Psora as the soil in which the seeds of Sycosis and Syphilis want to put down roots, the homœopathic treatment of chronic illness involves removing the soil so that there's nothing in which seeds can root or grow.

Understanding the theory of inherent predispositions to illness is as essential for effective progress assessment as it is for selecting the first and subsequent prescriptions. To effectively assess what is happening and why at any point, it is important to understand which inherent predisposition prevailed at what point in the patient's life and timeline of suffering. In that way, reappearing traces of inherent predispositions to illness during recovery are easily observed, and the reasons for their reappearance correctly understood.

Here's how the theory of inherent predispositions is applied in practice.

A patient's timeline of illness indicates that the slumbering under-productive recurring itching skin symptom predisposition 'Psora' was responsible for the symptoms that made them feel unwell for the first

---

[14] Dr. S. Hahnemann, *The Chronic Diseases: Their Peculiar Nature & Their Homœopathic Cure*

[15] Ibid

time. Some event or incident awakened it. The treatment received (not homœopathy) relieved some of the suffering but not all of the symptoms ever really went away completely. Later on, the original illness has changed. Different symptoms and conditions appeared. New symptoms—e.g. ulcerations, merge with the old symptoms; the new ulcerating symptoms belong to the destructive predisposition 'Syphilis'. The presence of a combination of predispositions complicates the illness. The patient becomes weaker. Later still, the suffering changes again. Completely different over growth of tissue symptoms appear signaling the presence of 'Sycosis.' Severely ill, the person presents for homœopathic treatment. In response to the correctly selected homœopathic medicine and dose the vital force regains power, begins rooting out traces of 'Psora'. The latest symptoms of the chronic illness are always the first to yield to treatment of Psora; but the oldest conditions and those that have been most constant and unchanged by previous treatment (among which are those that affect a particular region or part of the body) are the last to disappear. This only happens when all the remaining disorders have disappeared, and in all other respects the patient's health has been almost totally restored.

However, patient individuality and practitioner remedy and dose selection mistakes mean the ideal recovery scenario may not happen.

Application of the principle of inherent predispositions provides a useful context in which to understand what causes certain symptoms to appear at different times during life in response to prior treatment, as well as what to expect in response to homœopathic treatment. In that way we are we are not utterly bewildered by the recovery route the vital force takes a particular patient or the fleeting flare ups of symptoms associated with each predisposition. Practitioner ignorance of the *inherent predisposition to illness* principle creates the following obstacles to cure:

- Misperceiving chronic versus acute nature of an illness. [16]
- Ignorance about different treatment protocols for acute and chronic illness

---

[16] Dr. Samuel Hahnemann, *The Organon of Medicine*, Sixth edition, §72 – §78

- Incorrect characteristic symptom totality selection, imperfect remedy and dose selection, improper monitoring intervals, improper period for remedy repetition
- Failure to understand that acute flare-ups of a chronic condition, e.g. reappearance of an old skin eruption or joint pain, indicate reappearance of an inherent predisposition

The third fixed principle relates to the leading role *susceptibility* plays in illness and recovery.

Susceptibility: action and reaction

In the context of homœopathy, susceptibility is the degree of reactivity of our vital force. It is the quality or state of our vital force at any given moment. Our *vital force* and *susceptibility* are so integral and inseparable, it could be said that if the vital force is a face, then susceptibility is the expression on that face.

Hahnemann teaches that susceptibility is an unmistakable law of nature. It relates to how likely and to what degree we are mentally, emotionally and physically influenced by particular *inherent predispositions to illness*. As discussed previously, these predispositions dictate the degree to which the individual is influenced by circumstances, events, environments, internal and external changes, etc., and how slowly or quickly successful adjustment to those changes occurs.[17] Examples of stimuli to which we might react or be susceptible to in varying degrees include danger, heat, cold, light, darkness, food, offence, criticism, loss and lack or excess of love.

In health, we are susceptible to the things that enable us to thrive and able to resist harmful influences. We act and react proportionately, successfully and speedily adjusting to all manner of changes without missing a beat. For example, if it is cold we will turn on the heating, or add clothes almost automatically. When we are ill, a tiny draft of cold air affects us very deeply, and no matter how much we increase the heat

---

[17] Dr. S. Hahnemann, *Homœopathic Materia Medica Pura*

we just cannot get warm. There is a tendency towards becoming overwhelmed by a particular influence.

During the examination phase, patients narrate the history of their illness through their experience of symptoms. These experiences indicate not only the unique state of disturbance, but also the specific strength or weakness of the patient's vital force and susceptibility. Through this information, practitioners are able to determine the power and depth of the disturbance and the degree of resistance offered by the vital force.

Knowledge and application of the homœopathic principle of *Susceptibility* are important in another way. Health restoration produced by homœopathy takes place only because the individual is as susceptible to the homœopathic medicine and dose selected as they are to the illness. The greater the symptom-similarity between the symptoms of original natural illness experienced and the symptoms proved to have been induced by the homœopathic remedy, the less homœopathic medicine is required and the quicker we may remove that patient's susceptibility to that particular suffering.

Failure to understand or apply the principle of susceptibility leads to selection of improper medicinal doses. Incorrect doses create the obstacle of unnecessarily overstimulating the vital force, inducing it to overreact to medicines and doses. The patient experiences intensification of *original natural* symptoms and/or appearance of uncomfortable, unnatural symptoms. Symptoms that were never part of the original illness are now among the symptoms experienced. Where there is an intermingling of natural, original symptoms with the appearance of 'unnatural' or medicinal symptoms, there is extreme practitioner confusion about exactly what is to be treated. The homœopathic *Materia Medica*, the medicine knowledge base, provides clarity. Under the medicine given, look for the new symptoms. If they are listed, this confirms the medicine has the proven power to produce those symptoms. Therefore, the medicine was well chosen but the dose was ill chosen. If the new symptoms are not listed, both medicine and dose were unsuitable. A reanalysis of the case is required.

In chronic illness, to disregard patient susceptibility and prevailing strength of the vital force and routinely start treatment with the most powerful doses risks severe injury to the vital force. It exposes patients to avoidable, severe and often intolerable intensification of suffering. It demonstrates practitioner ignorance of the fact that, in homœopathy, no dose of the correct medicine is too weak or too small to effect a change or cure, and the gentlest, proper dose is always the smallest minimal dose.

Totality of characteristic individualising symptoms

The fourth fixed principle governing homœopathic practice is the *Totality of Characteristic Individualising Symptoms*. This relates to the removal and annihilation of the disease in its whole extent. For the cure of every disease, the totality of characteristic symptoms must be removed[18]; the symptom totality indicates the correct homœopathic medicine for that purpose. To cure, the true practitioner of homœopathy must view the illness in its entirety rather than focusing on single symptoms and separate parts. This means that those seeking homœopathic treatment must be willing to think deeply and present the full history of their illness. In that way, the remedy with the proven power to induce the greatest number of characteristic symptoms similar to the complete illness experienced will be selected, recovery will start to occur and be sustained.

Success in the selection of the most symptom-similar medicine depends entirely on the view of illness taken by a practitioner. As this outlook varies, so does the chance of success. Through the symptoms the vital force produces, a portrait of the illness is painted for both patient and practitioner. The aim of all practitioners is to realise an undistorted view of the illness in its totality. This is achieved through considering each person with all their symptoms and creating a complete, multidimensional portrait rather than a one-sided view.

---

[18] Dr. S. Hahnemann, *The Organon of Medicine* Sixth edition, §7

Practitioner failure to understand or rigorously apply this principle will have a devastating effect on patients.

> The oftener you prescribe for different groups of symptoms the worse it is for your patient, because it tends to rivet the constitutional state upon the patient and to make him incurable. Do not prescribe until you have found the remedy that is similar to the whole case, even though it is clear in your mind that one remedy may be more similar to one particular group of symptoms and another remedy to another group.[19]

To underline the range of distorted views taken by practitioners, here are a few examples:

- A practitioner who views cases only from the pathological aspect, or a patient's temperament; eye or hair colour; a patient's complexion, or height
- A practitioner whose view comprises of either only keynote symptoms of certain medicines memorised, or the opinion of some other practitioner
- A practitioner who observes the totality as an alternating state —one set of symptoms one time and a different set another time after a change has occurred—rather than considering them all to be part of the whole.

This last example leads to changes of remedies with every shift in the illness, but at the end of the year the patient has grown steadily worse. Unfortunately, in these cases, the practitioner will conclude that each group of symptoms has been 'cured'. This type of work is a failure because the practitioner has not viewed the patient from the totality of symptoms. Carelessness in selecting and considering the symptoms after they have been recorded in the history taking leads to indifferent results.[20]

One thing that is often not accepted or understood by prescribers of homœopathic medicines is that homœopathy is only useful in the removal of symptoms produced *naturally* during illness. It is unable to remove symptoms of iatrogenic diseases, side-effect symptoms caused

---

[19] Dr. J. T. Kent, *Lectures on Homœopathic Philosophy*

[20]*Kent's, New Remedies, Clinical Cases, Lesser Writings, Aphorisms & Precepts*, compiled by Dr. W.W. Sherwood

by routine, prolonged and frequently repeated strong doses of mainstream medicines. Therefore, to find the correct homœopathic medicine, the practitioner must discriminate carefully between the origins of symptoms experienced by the patient as their story unfolds. Those that are symptoms of *natural* disease are retained and used for homœopathic medicine selection. Symptoms that occur in response to medication are excluded. They tend to disappear gradually once the drug that produced them is discontinued. The clearest image of the illness that can be given is when the patient began to feel unwell for the very first time and is able to describe the first symptoms that appeared before mainstream medicine or other treatments were administered and altered the original state of illness. Those original symptoms of the original illness represent the disease that is to be cured.

Viewing a single person to be in several different states at the same time, and treating each symptom or condition separately with several different medicines is not the homœopathic view of illness. It is the view of illness and what is to be treated taken by ordinary medicine. Another distorted view occurs when a practitioner takes a few symptoms randomly or every single symptom the patient has experienced in their life.

This is how it should be done:

- The totality of symptoms and its corresponding symptom-similar homœopathic medicine are both based on the same idea
- The totality is related equally to the medicine and to the disease. The symptoms of the remedy must correspond to the symptoms experienced during the disease.

In examining each case of illness, the homœopathic practitioner obtains what appears to the novice to be a heterogeneous mass of symptoms, or fragments of symptoms. Sometimes the patient's report may not appear to include even one complete symptom. Instead, the perceptible symptoms of disease are often broken up and scattered throughout the different parts of the patient's organism. The practitioner finds a clearly expressed sensation in some part, but without any accompanying worsening or ameliorating modifying condition. In another part, the practitioner finds a clearly expressed worsening or ameliorating condition, but an indefinite sensation is found; or perhaps the patient will simply report feeling better or worse under certain conditions. In reality the patient is expressing incomplete symptoms, only parts of very few complete symptoms, which the examiner must bring together to complete a picture of the whole suffering.

Hahnemann instructs true practitioners of homœopathy to recognise that the totality of the disease symptoms and the disease itself [21] are the same thing and clearly articulates the significance of taking the symptom-image totality view of illness rather than any other view. According to Hahnemann, it is only the more *striking, singular rare uncommon and peculiar,* (characteristic) signs and symptoms that provide the unique portrait of an individual's totality of suffering,[22] that are to be compared with symptoms of medicinal substances recorded in the homœopathic database of tested medicines. This view of illness underpins the correct thought process required to find the correct remedy.

In Hahnemann's pure homœopathic healing art, it is the *patient as a whole* who is sick, rather than his head, or her eye or heart. For example, if there is a stitching pain felt in the eye, the type of pain belongs to the eye, which belongs to the individual, and the sensation 'stitching pain in the eye' is noted as a characteristic symptom of this particular patient and their eye. If walking increases the eye pain, 'eye pain worse by walking' is noted as a characteristic aggravation of the eye symptom.

> The totality eliminates all theoretical elements and the speculations of traditional medicine and deals only with the actual manifest facts. The facts it assembles, are not according to some arbitrary or imaginary form, but according to a natural order.[23]

During the patient examination, the most important illness descriptions are those that provide characteristic individualising information that makes that case unique. A 'characteristic

---

[21] Dr. S. Hahnemann, *The Organon of Medicine*, Sixth edition §17

[22] Ibid §153

[23] Dr. H. A. Roberts, Annie C. Wilson, *Introduction to Boenninghausen's Therapeutic Pocketbook*

individualising' symptom has several components: causation, location, sensation, sides, time and extension. A symptom with all components is called a 'complete' characteristic symptom. When trying to discriminate between symptoms the more complete a symptom is, the more it characterises the patient, the more useful it is for finding the correct medicine.

Characteristic symptoms are also essential for accurate potency selection. Cure using homœopathy requires sufficient vital force susceptibility to the medicine. There must not only be shared symptom-similarity between symptoms produced by medicines and symptoms produced naturally during illness, but also shared similarity between the dose of medicine and vital force susceptibility. Where the symptoms of a case are not clearly developed and there is an absence or scarcity of characteristic symptoms, an imperfect choice of medicine is very likely, to which the vital force will be less susceptible. Less vital force susceptibility indicates a less potent dose of a medicine is required so as to avoid overwhelming it. However, when the characteristic symptoms of a case correspond very closely to the characteristic symptoms produced by a medicine, patient susceptibility to the medicine is considered to be higher, requiring consideration of medium to high potency doses.

Let's say the patient reports 'itching'. The proficient practitioner knows that is pretty useless information. It won't lead to the correct medicine. So she formulates open questions, for example 'tell me more about the itching.' Gradually the common symptom 'itching' is transformed by the patient's words into the characteristic symptom: skin itching from insect bites, worse at night, worse from getting wet, better scratching until it bleeds.

This type of high-quality patient information makes using the homœopathic Repertory, which is an index of symptoms and their corresponding medicines, so much quicker and efficient.

In the hierarchical remedy selection method, to provide a coherent consistent framework or skeleton upon which and around which to build the *Totality of Characteristic Individualising Symptoms* structure, information is organised and prioritised under these headings:

Causation(s) where known with certainty and without speculation

Striking, Singular, Uncommon, Peculiar characteristic signs and symptoms: things that make you hesitate and meditate, e.g. menstrual flow only at night

General Mental Disposition and modifying features

General Physical Disposition and modifying features

Particulars: region, affinity, location, extensions and modifying features

Sensations and modifying features[24]

These components form the symptom image totality portrait that represents the spirit, mind and body disturbance experienced. Due to the uniqueness of each case of illness, the patient examination may not provide information for all sections. Don't worry. It is not the quantity of symptoms that indicates the correct homœopathic medicine; it is the quality of individualising symptoms identified and chosen for the prescription basis. The symptom totality individualises the disturbance, combines knowledge of disease with what is known, through experiment, to be curative in medicines. It is a 'mug-shot' that directs us straight to the symptom-similar medicine for that particular person in that particular characteristic state of disorder. Viewing the symptom totality correctly as Hahnemann instructs, improves the opportunity for rapid, gentle permanent recovery. Practitioners seldom use it now. Not because it is inefficient, but because it demands intelligent, fine discrimination between which symptoms should be included in the totality and which should be excluded.

Application of those four fixed principles provides knowledge of what causes and indicates disease, exactly what must be treated and the prevailing strength or weakness of the individual's vital force.

---

[24] Dr. J. T. Kent, *Repertory of the Homœopathic Materia Medica*

If you haven't already done so, it's time to pause, relax the brain muscle for a while, perhaps stretch your legs have a cup of tea and a biscuit, then continue.

The following fixed principles are at the heart of homœopathy:

- Smallest dose: dilution and potentiation
- Know the curative power of each individual medicine
- Let likes be cured with likes
- Proper dose: single substance, single dose

Rooted in the branch of medical science known as *Materia Medica*— which studies the history, preparation, properties and effects upon the living system, in health and disease, of all the various therapeutic substances[25]—these principles remind us that all medicines have as much power to harm as they do to heal and, therefore, must always be used judiciously.

Smallest dose: dilution and potentiation

The fifth fixed fundamental principle of homœopathy is crucial to gentle cure, but is often singled out by our detractors as proof that homœopathy is unscientific. It is easy to why they would come to that conclusion. Most medical scientists view the universe through the principle of materialism: the theory or belief that nothing exists except matter and its movements and modifications. They may not know that as stated earlier, homœopathy is a medical system based on the principle of vitalism, the theory that the origin and phenomena of life are dependent on a force or principle distinct from purely chemical or physical forces. If medical science knew of the theory of vitalism and that the pharmacological process of dilution and potentiation of medicinal substances used in homœopathy is based on a fundamental principle of the universe often applied in physics: 'the quantity of

---

[25] Dr. John B. Beck, *Lectures on Materia Medica and Therapeutics*

action necessary to effect any change in nature is the least possible,'[26] the pharmacology used in homœopathy would be easier to perceive as scientific.

To really get to grips with smallest dose principle it is necessary to understand that the homœopathic principle of cure through shared similitude between symptoms experienced naturally during illness and symptoms produced by medicines is useless without the dilution and potentiation medicine preparation process, because it is through the vehicle of infinitesimal medicinal doses that homœopathy avoids everything that might weaken the patient or cause pain in the slightest degree, and at the same time assists the ailing vital force of nature in the most harmless way.

Homœopathy harnesses the innate life preserving, self recovery capacity of the human body, which continuously, automatically, unconsciously exerts an effort to remain intact and whole. Instinctively the body offers resistance to everything that tends to disturb its normal functioning. That resistance is experienced in uncomfortable changes, sensations and conditions such as pain, fever inflammation, and changed secretions and excretions, etc. The partly psychical, partly physical, natural conflicting forces to which the human body is exposed do not possess the power of unconditionally morbidly deranging our health. They only make us ill when we are sufficiently disposed and susceptible and our vital force is weakened. Hence, exposure to natural inimical forces does not produce disease in everyone nor at all times.[27]

Through experiment Hahnemann discovered ingestion or application of medicines has an entirely different effect. He found that the living human body is much more disposed to let its health be altered by the vastly superior power of medicines, than the inferior power of natural illness. Experience has proven incontestably that medicines possess an absolute unconditional superior power to disrupt health. Every medicine acts at *all* times, under *all* circumstances, on every living human being, and if the dose is large enough it will

[26]Pierre-Louis Maupertius 1698–1759 French Mathematician and Philosopher

[27] Dr. S. Hahnemann, *The Organon of Medicine* Sixth edition, Author's Preface

produce its own peculiar distinctly noticeable symptoms. Which is certainly not the case with natural diseases.[28]

Depending on the quantity of the substance or the power of drug dose, the action of a drug may produce suffering or cure. There is a so-called primary action and secondary reaction of drugs. The primary action elicits one group of symptoms, whereas the secondary action elicits a directly opposite set of symptoms. For example, a physiological dose of opium produces symptoms of deep sleep or diarrhoea in the primary action, and long lasting wakefulness or constipation in the secondary reaction. Practitioners of the ordinary medical system which is based on the principle of materialism, argues that human beings are only affected by physiological doses of crude substances where molecules of the original substance remain. Their objective is always to produce a direct, definite, predetermined physiological effect on the body. To be therapeutic a drug must produce symptoms that are *opposite* to the illness symptoms experienced: *anti-inflammatory, anti-septic, anti-biotic, anti-coagulant*, etc. The physiological size and strength of the dose is always the *maximum* consistent with safety and patient age. Bodily resistance experienced as extra suffering or 'side effects', is considered to be peculiar and worth tolerating because the benefits of a drug are perceived to outweigh its disadvantages.

Rooted in the principle of vitalism, homœopathy perceives the appearance of symptoms to signal a disturbance of the vital force of nature which is responding to conflicting forces causing it to struggle to preserve life. The object of homœopathic treatment is never to produce symptoms, but to remove them completely in a direct manner.[29] As the effects of the well-chosen medicine resemble the experience of the symptom totality, medicine and dose encounter little or no protective bodily resistance. To be therapeutic, the ideal homœopathic medicinal dose is one that is so small that at best the symptom disappears, or at worst it is only capable of producing a slight

---

[28] Dr. S. Hahnemann, *Materia Medica Pura; The Organon of Medicine*, Sixth edition, §30, §32, §33.

[29] This is done by selecting the smallest dose possible of a natural substance that when administered to <u>healthy</u> humans in experiments, has been proven to be capable of producing the greatest number of symptoms *similar* to those experienced by the patient.

temporary intensification of the *characteristic symptoms,* and not large enough to produce a severe intensification of those symptoms or new different symptoms.

To heal gently, calm, strengthen and encourage the weakened vital force to restore order as rapidly as possible, the healing properties of crude natural substances must be released in the most harmless way. Then they must be specially adapted to influence the intangible vital force without overwhelming it. The medicinal substances must be:

- Pure in quality

- Non-toxic

- Incapable of producing unwanted side effect symptoms.

- Soluble in water and alcohol

- Infinitesimal in quantity

- Easily accessible to the ever changing, distressed intangible vital force

- Capable of being instantly appropriated by the sentient nerves and assimilable by the whole body

Hahnemann observed that the human body responds differently to large and small drug doses. For example, a teaspoon of Ipecacuanha causes sickness and vomiting; however, under certain conditions, only drop-doses of Ipecacuanha are required to cure sickness and vomiting. Large doses of opium bind up the bowels, while a small dose loosens them.

The purpose of the peculiar homœopathic medicine preparation process is as follows:

- To render crude, inert, virulent or poisonous substances into less harmful, more soluble, and assimilable

- To liberate and expose the most subtle essence of the medicinal substance and its power

- To create the smallest dose of medicine capable of curing

- To moderate the strength of the medicine in some degree, while increasing the medicine's power to penetrate into the body

- To ensure each dose penetrates the body more deeply, but with less disruption to the vital force than the previous one.

To achieve all those goals, Hahnemann experimented for several years and formulated the homœopathic 'dilution and potentiation' medicine preparation method: a mathematically precise scale of substance measurement, serial division, trituration, dilution and agitation. In this pharmacological process, the smallest unit of matter is serially divided into separate particles and diluted in certain definite proportions of parts of a natural substance to parts of a non-medicinal fresh milk sugar vehicle. The medicinal substance is distributed equally between each particle, through prolonged mechanical serial trituration (friction, grinding and rubbing) in a mortar with a pestle, six times triturating for six minutes, six times scraping together for four minutes. The triturated, diluted medicinal powder is rendered soluble by mixing it in a vial with definite proportions of distilled water and alcohol. The vial is then "potentiated" shaken vigorously with the brachial force of two downward strokes of the arm. The vial label should state that the contents have been shaken twice, the date, the substance name and potency. A definite number of pellets is moistened with a medicinal liquid, dried quickly and put into another vial ready for dosing. Hahnemann states:

> Not only do these medicinal substances develop their powers in prodigious degree, they also change their physiochemical demeanour, in such a way that whereas before in their crude form no one could ever perceive any solubility in alcohol or water, after this peculiar transmutation they become wholly soluble in water as well as alcohol.[30]

Hahnemann describes the complete homœopathic medicine preparation method in detail in The Medicines section of *Chronic Diseases: Their Peculiar Nature and Their Homœopathic Cure.*

---

[30]Dr. S. Hahnemann, *The Chronic Diseases: Their Peculiar Nature & Their Homœopathic Cure*

Hahnemann's 'centesimal' potency scale of homœopathic medicine, (1-part medicinal substance to 99 parts of inert non-medicinal diluting medium, to give a ratio of 1:100), is always mathematically serially diluted and vigorously shaken with *two* downward strokes of the arm rather than the ten strokes given by other practitioners. After many experiments and searching comparison with patients, Hahnemann says he preferred to give only two strokes because the double shake increases the quantity of the medicinal forces developed, like the ten downward shakes, but not in as high a degree. Therefore, the two downward stroke potency achieves a weaker—although somewhat more highly potentised and more penetrating medicine—than the dose using ten shakes.[31] This way, each dose penetrates the body more deeply, but with less disruption to the vital force than the previous one.

Each dose of homœopathic medicine is selected according to the 'potency' perceived by the prescriber to be the smallest dose sufficient to induce longlasting recovery without harming the vital force.

A dose may be administered either orally by mouth dissolving the pellet on the tongue, or nasally by holding a vial containing a medicine up to the nostrils. Administration of homœopathic medicines this way, where the medicine enters the body through the sensory nerves of the olfactory system, is especially useful in the treatment of unconscious individuals.

After many years in clinical practice using centesimal potencies up to 30c, Hahnemann observed the following:

- Sometimes in the treatment of chronic illness, a single dose of an appropriately selected homœopathic remedy completes cure only slowly, although progressively, within 40, 50, 60, or 100 days.
- That there might be a way to halve recovery time.
- That centesimal potencies prepared using a powerful agitation machine, act almost immediately, but with furious, even dangerous, violence—especially in weak patients.

---

[31] Ibid

- That overreaction always occurs when a homœopathic medicine is repeated in the same unmodified dose, especially in rapidly repeated doses.[32]

This final point is true because the stricken vital force doesn't accept unchanged doses without resistance. This is experienced by the appearance of symptoms that are different from the original existing similar symptoms being treated. Such resistance happens because the first dose of medicine changed the original state of the vital force. Therefore, a second similar dose of the same medicine no longer finds the vital force in the same condition it was before the first dose, and thus, the reaction will be different. By receiving another unchanged dose, the patient may be made sick in another way—or even made sicker than he was. By now, only those symptoms the medicine is capable of producing—those that were not similar to the original disease—remain active. This being the case, no step towards cure can follow, only a further aggravation of the patient's condition.[33] Patients may have to suffer days or weeks for the medicinal symptoms to gradually subside. Intervention with selection and administration of antidotal medicines might be needed to calm things down. A previously simple case becomes unnecessarily complicated.

Around 1836-7 Hahnemann began to experiment and counter-experiment to perfect the medicinal preparations, to halve recovery time, eliminate the obstacles to gentle recovery mentioned above, and benefit the most severely ill and weakest individuals. Five years later he changed the standard preparation method, created the '50-millesimal' potency scale, and described it in the sixth final edition of *The Organon of Medicine* sections §269–§272. In the new method, the ratio of parts of medicinal substance to diluent increases from 1:100 (centesimal scale), to 1:50,000. To increase the power of penetration into the body with even less disruption of the vital force, he increased the number of agitations of the vial from two powerful downward strokes of the arm to 8, 10, or 12 powerful strokes, this time against a hard but elastic body

---

[32] Dr. S. Hahnemann, *The Organon of Medicine*, Sixth edition,§246, §247,

[33] Dr. S. Hahnemann, *The Organon of Medicine*, Sixth edition, §246, §247, §270 F/n 155

such as a leather-bound book. Hahnemann says 'At the end of four of five years I found it to be the most powerful and at the same time mildest in action, i.e. as the most perfected...'[34]

Always provided the most symptom-similar medicine is chosen, curative changes induced in response to LM/Q doses tend to be quicker and deeper, yet gentler and last longer than those induced by centesimal doses. Should an LM/Q potency dosing patient experience symptom intensification, they need only stop dosing immediately and the intensified symptoms will rapidly disappear on their own, usually within a few hours rather than over days or weeks. In response to well-chosen remedies administered strictly according to Hahnemann's LM/Q dosing protocols, homœopathic patients tend to walk steadily and continuously up a gentle slope towards complete recovery. LM/Q dosing patients are more likely to achieve the highest ideal of cure: rapid, gentle and permanent restoration of health, or removal and annihilation of the disease in its whole extent, in the shortest, most reliable and most harmless way...[35]

Even though the LM/Q dosing method surpasses the centesimal method in terms of power, gentleness, reduction of overreaction and shortening recovery time, the LM/Q potency scale is not used widely. Although Hahnemann described it fully in the Sixth edition of *The Organon of Medicine*, that final edition was not published until 1921. By then some practitioners considered it necessary to increase the centesimal potency scale beyond the 30c potency and introduced different methods of dilution and potentiation and machinery to develop higher centesimal potencies: 1M, 10M, 50M CM, MM, etc. The precision afforded by the LM/Q dosinging method in terms of adapting medicinal dose to the needs of each patient's vital force is overlooked. The most popular potency and dosing method is still the centesimal scale.

As discussed above the *Smallest dose: dilution and potentiation* homœopathic principle attracts most controversy, ridicule and

---

[34] Ibid, §270, Footnote 156

[35] Dr. S. Hahnemann, *The Organon of Medicine*, §2

scepticism due to the failure of medical scientists to recognise that homœopathy is based on the theory of vitalism, rather than materialism. According to materialistic medical science the human body remains unaffected by dilutions of substances that do not contain even one molecule of the original substance, such as homœopathic potencies above 12c. If that were true, how may we explain the experience of individuals who participated in Hahnemann's experiments to discover exactly which symptoms each medicine is capable of producing in healthy people reporting so many symptoms after ingesting 30c doses of homœopathic medicines?

Hahnemann also suggests prejudice against the smallness of homœopathic doses exists because:

> First, the skeptic is ignorant of the fact that by means of grinding each substance to a fine powder the internal medicinal power is wonderfully developed and is, as it were, liberated from its material bonds by that process. With the result it operates more penetratingly and more freely upon the human body.

> Second, the skeptics purely arithmetical mind believes that it sees in the homœopathic medicine preparation process nothing more than example of enormous subdivision, a mere material division and imitation in which, as every child knows, every part must be less than the whole. The skeptic does not observe, that in elevating the internal medicinal power of the substance beyond material physical levels, the material receptacle of these natural forces is not taken into consideration at all.

> Third, the skeptic has no experience in connection with the action of such powerful medicinal preparations.[36]

To ignore the 'least medicine is best medicine' purpose of homœopathy is to fail to take into account that recovery from illness using homœopathy cannot occur unless there is similarity between a)the existing characteristic individualising symptoms experienced, b)the symptoms a particular medicine has the power to induce in healthy people, and c)similitude between prevailing potency of the patient's vital force and potency of the medicinal dose.

---

[36] Dr. S. Hahnemann, *The Lesser Writings of Samuel Hahnemann*

Other reasons that indicate only the smallest dose of homœopathic medicine is required to induce cure are:

- The individual is susceptible to outside influences
- The individual's sufferings indicate the illness has penetrated beyond the body's natural defences
- The higher the potency, the less toxicity and greater the purity of the medicinal substance
- There is no bodily resistance to the homœopathic remedy

A vital component of homœopathic practice is knowledge of the most suitable mode of medicine preparation, the quantity required to induce cure and proper period for repeating the dose. Hahnemann urges his followers to avoid prejudice towards or against particular medicines or potencies.

The next fixed principle relates to gathering knowledge about which symptoms are produced by which medicinal substance.

The curative power of each individual medicine

Medicinal substances are not dead masses in the ordinary sense of the term; their true essential nature is pure force. Before we can hope to be able to find and select a medicine capable of producing the greatest number of symptoms as similar as possible to the totality of the symptoms of the natural disease to be cured, all the morbid symptoms and alterations in health that each of them is specially capable of developing in the healthy individual must first have been observed.[37] Therefore, in homœopathy, before administering medicines to *sick* people, it is critical that we investigate and gather accurate information about how each individual medicine affects *healthy* people.

To achieve this goal Hahnemann formulated a methodology to ensure purity of the experiments, so that the true effects of each medicinal substance might be clearly expressed. The experiments were

---

[37]Dr. S. Hahnemann, *The Organon of Medicine*, Sixth edition, §106 – §108.

performed on males and females who were as healthy as possible, and under regulated external conditions as nearly alike as possible. He administered doses according to the centesimal potency preparation method. Experience taught him low (3c–12c) potencies produce only the more general symptoms common to many medicines. To clearly differentiate between medicines, Hahnemann wanted to elicit the specific characteristic symptoms peculiar to each medicine. So he chose the infinitesimal moderate potency: 30c[38] even though it is doubtful that any molecules of the original substance remain in such a dose, and administered it in dry pellet doses of *natural* substances to both male and female *healthy* people, two doses daily[39] until they began to experience mental, emotional or physical signs of discomfort, which they noted down. A medium potency is enough to produce the greatest amount of characteristic symptoms but not enough to induce lasting effects. The medicinal symptoms rapidly disappear by themselves once repetition of dosing stops at the end of the experiment. To ensure purity of data gathered:

As the experimenter cannot, any more than any other human being, be absolutely and perfectly healthy, should slight ailments to which she was liable before the start of the experiment reappear during the experiment, those ailments must be placed between brackets, to indicate they are dubious and cannot be confirmed as solely derived from the medicine under investigation.[40]

The experimenter must possess a sufficient amount of intelligence to be able to express and describe his sensations in accurate terms.[41]

If the person cannot write, the physician must be informed by him every day of what has occurred to him, and how it took place. What is noted down as authentic information on this point, however, must be chiefly the voluntary narration of the person who makes the experiment, nothing conjectural and as little as possible derived from answers to leading questions admitted; everything must be ascertained with the same caution as I have counselled

---

[38] Dr. S. Hahnemann *Materia Medica Pura*

[39] Ibid

[40] Dr. S. Hahnemann, *Materia Medica Pura,*

[41] Dr. S. Hahnemann, *The Organon of Medicine* Sixth edition, §126

above (§84–§99) for the investigation of the phenomena and for tracing the picture of natural diseases.[42]

To eliminate the potential for bias, the name of the substance under investigation was withheld from drug-trial participants. At the end of every day during an experiment, all participants were interviewed separately. Each symptom experienced was meticulously recorded, including the name of each participant against each symptom experienced. All the symptoms documented during the experiment were collated. Among those substances tested, Carbo Vegetalis (charcoal) induced 720 symptoms and Belladonna 1,440 symptoms. The first phase of Hahnemann's experiments involved testing sixty-seven pure natural substances. His clinical trials provided not only invaluable evidence of the character and intensity of mental, emotional and physical illness that a particular natural substance has the power to induce in healthy people, but most importantly how even the smallest medicinal dose, in dilutions far exceeding 12c, is enough to affect the human body and induce illness.

To provide sufficient homœopathic medicines, Hahnemann continued experimenting with different natural medicinal substances throughout his life, but not on animals. He understood that human beings are more similar to one another than they are to animals, and that the vital operations and processes of animal and human bodies differ. He was also aware that disease manifests itself in all spheres of the body: mental, emotional and physical. Human experimenters cannot accurately record the subjective feelings of animals when animals cannot communicate their subjective feelings to humans. This explains why treatment of animals using homœopathy is more difficult.

Let likes be cured with likes

This principle is the fundamental tenet of homœopathic practice. Hahnemann's experience with medicines taught him that *natural* disease is different from artificial, medicinal disease. Natural disease is

[42] Ibid §140

conditional upon the individual being sufficiently disposed or susceptible to powerful, partly psychological, partly physical, external harmful influences.[43] Hahnemann gained knowledge about the symptoms each medicinal dose produces in healthy people through his earliest experiments conducted on himself. He took four drachms of cinchona bark twice a day, which induced paroxysms of chills and fever. When he observed patients in his medical practice experiencing similar symptoms, he administered a dose of cinchona bark and noted that the symptoms disappeared.

Continuing his medical research, Hahnemann posed the question: is it possible to cure disease through the principle of shared symptom-similarity between medicines and illnesses? He discovered that for homœopathic medicines to effect a cure, they must first be capable of producing in the human body symptoms of an *artificial* disease as *similar* as possible to the disease to be cured, and second be administered in a dose that is somewhat more powerful than the power of the original natural disease. Although the *artificial* disease caused by the medicine is stronger than the natural disease, it is much more easily overcome by the vital force because it is only a simulation, an *artificial manifestation of the natural disease.*

In experiments resembling Phase Two clinical trials, in which a drug is given to people who have a medical condition to see if it does indeed help them, Hahnemann noted the characteristic individualising symptoms experienced by a sick person, and searched the experimental data for a medicine proven to induce the greatest number of similar symptoms in healthy people. He observed that after taking infrequent infinitesimal sub-physiological doses of such medicines, sick people rapidly regained health.

Hahnemann concluded that:

A medicine which, in its action of the healthy human body, has demonstrated its power of producing the greatest number of symptoms similar to this observable in the case of disease under treatment, does also, in doses of suitable potency and attenuation, rapidly radically and

---

[43] Dr. S. Hahnemann, The *Organon of Medicine,* Fourth edition Author's Preface; The *Organon of Medicine* Sixth edition, §31

permanently remove the totality of the symptoms…that is to say (§6 – §16), the whole disease present, and change it into health; and that all medicines cure, without exception, those diseases whose symptoms most nearly resemble their own, and leave none of them uncured.[44]

This depends on the following homœopathic law of nature: A weaker dynamic affection is permanently extinguished in the living organism by a stronger one, if the latter while differing in kind is very similar to the former in its manifestations.[45]

…Without causing pain or weakening, they just suffice to remove the natural malady whence this result: that without weakening, injuring or torturing him in the very least, the natural disease is extinguished, and the patient, even while he is getting better, gains in strength and thus is cured…[46]

His experiments with medicines and people verified the homœopathic law of nature, *The Law of Similars*: cure through shared symptom-similarity between medicine and illness is possible. Hahnemann had achieved his goal of rapidly curing disease in the gentlest, least harmful way.

Lack of attention to the exact words used in the Law of Similars, has led to a continuing distortion of homœopathy.

The dictionary definition of the word 'similar' is 'having a resemblance in appearance, character or quantity, without being identical'. The dictionary definition of the word 'same' is: 'identical; not different.' Where the word 'similar' is accidentally or deliberately replaced by the word 'same', instantly the medical practice of homœopathy is transformed into the medical practice of isopathy: the ancient theory of using morbid products of a disease for the cure of the same disease [*Aequalia aequalibus*], or curing a sick person's diseased organ by instructing them to eat the analogous organ of a healthy animal. Mainstream medical practice uses isopathy to confer temporary artificial immunity from certain diseases by inoculating individuals with identical viruses of those diseases. The etymological distortion by some

---

[44] Dr. S. Hahnemann, *The Organon of Medicine*, Sixth edition, §25.

[45] Dr. S. Hahnemann, *The Organon of Medicine*, Sixth edition, §26

[46] Dr. S. Hahnemann, *The Organon of Medicine*, Sixth edition, Author's Preface.

prescribers to replace the word 'similar' with the word 'same,' has allowed treatment of symptoms of a particular disease with medicines made from substances secreted in the course of that disease, to be considered as homœopathy, which plainly it is not.

Homœopathy cures using medicinal substances that are *always different in kind and nature* from the illness or that which causes the illness but produce effects resembling the symptoms of illness experienced. Hahnemann states clearly:

> The homœopathic system of medicine never pretended to cure a disease by the *same*, the *identical* agent by which the disease was produced–this has been inculcated on the unintelligent opponents often enough but, as it seems, in vain:–no! it only cures by means of any agent never exactly corresponding to, never *identical* with the cause of the disease, but by means of a medicine that, possess the peculiar power of being able to produce only a *similar* morbid state, and this is the mode most in conformity with nature.[47]

> Without this difference in the nature of the morbid affection from that of the medicinal affection, a cure was impossible; if the two were not merely of a similar, but of the same nature, consequently identical, then no result (or only an aggravation of the malady) would ensue; as for example, if we were to touch a chancre with other chancre poison, a cure would never result therefrom.[48]

Consequently, where there is shared similitude between symptoms produced naturally by the illness and symptoms produced by the medicine, Hahnemann recommends treating symptoms of the venereal diseases Syphilis with homœopathic preparations made from Mercury, and Gonorrhoea with medicines made from the leaves of the plant Thuja Occidentalis.

Proper dose: single substance, single dose

After selecting the relevant symptom-similar medicine, the next task is to give careful consideration to how much and how often the patient

[47] Dr. S. Hahnemann, *Materia Medica Pura,*

[48] Dr. S. Hahnemann, *Materia Medica Pura,*

should receive the medicine. This principle states that to restore health, the proper dose of homœopathic medicine is always a single substance in the smallest, single dose, given as infrequently as possible.

Hahnemann's instructions on the proper dose explodes another myth about homœopathy: that any dose of homœopathic medicine administered according to any number of repetitions at any interval will produce a curative response. Creators of that myth fail to understand that dosage is a key part of the homœopathic medical doctrine. The medicinal dose selected is required to achieve a delicate balance: it must be sufficient to assist the weakened vital force of nature but insufficient to induce overreaction or snuff the vital force out entirely. Failure to understand the importance of the proper dose leads to endless improper changes of medicines, unnecessary complication of very simple cases and avoidable patient misery.

In homœopathic practice, the optimal minimal dose is individually tailored specifically to the unique needs of each person and their illness. Cure depends on accurate selection of both medicine and potency.[49] Diligent practitioners avoid bias against a particular potency scale. Whether the potency selected in centesimal or LM/Q, the goal is always similitude between a patient's prevailing strength, illness and medicinal symptoms. You never know whether you have succeeded until the patient responds. The balance of dose and frequency is crucial: too large a dose and the vital force will produce an intolerable, damaging overreaction, too frequent and the curative response is interrupted.

Too frequent centesimal dosing is a common error often caused by dependence on information contained in the fifth rather than Sixth edition of *The Organon of Medicine* and ignorance of the fact that, in homœopathy, it is the minimal dose that effects cure rather than the maximal dose. Even if the first dose proves beneficial, a second or third unaltered dose would not prove to be beneficial, because:

> The vital principle does not accept such unchanged doses without resistance, that is, without other symptoms of the medicine manifesting themselves

---

[49] Dr. S. Hahnemann, *The Organon of Medicine*, Sixth edition, §275.

than those similar to the disease to be cured, because the former dose has already accomplished the expected change in the vital principle, and a second dynamically wholly similar, unchanged dose of the same medicine no longer finds, therefore, the same conditions of the vital force. The patient may indeed be made sick in another way by receiving other such unchanged doses, even sicker than he was, for now only those symptoms of the given remedy remain active, which were not homœopathic to the original disease, hence no step towards cure can follow, only a true aggravation of the condition of the patient.[50]

Here are two practitioner created divergences from the Proper Dose rule:

- **Pluralist**: This method is based on the idea that there is more than a single disease to treat in each patient, therefore more than one medicine at a time is given. Often a medium potency (12c-15c) is given daily, with a lower potency (6X)[51] of an "organ" specific remedy given in the morning for "drainage," then a high potency (30c) nosode[52] given on the weekend.
- **Complexist**: This method combines several medicines into a single dose, which is given, often daily.

To avoid injury, a homœopathic medicine is never routinely administered repeatedly without patient review in between doses to confirm that the first dose of remedy selected was beneficial, and another dose is definitely required.

When medicine dose and vital force are in harmony, the curative response is both breathtaking and unforgettable for patient and practitioner. You get to observe and appreciate the genius of homœopathy. Prescribing with that accuracy demands great skill. According to Hahnemann, the correct minimal dose is a single substance, a single medicine, in a single dose.

---

[50]Dr. S. Hahnemann, *The Organon of Medicine,* Sixth edition §247; F/n 133

[51]The X designation refers to a potency scale dilution divergence from Hahnemann's medicine preparation method.

[52] A medicine prepared from a substance secreted in the course of a disease.

In no case under treatment is it necessary and therefore not permissible to administer to a patient more than one single, simple medicinal substance at one time. It is inconceivable how the slightest doubt could exist regarding whether it was more consistent with nature and more rational to prescribe a single, simple medicine at one time in a disease or a mixture of several differently acting drugs. It is absolutely not allowed in homœopathy, the one true, simple and natural art of healing, to give a patient at one time two different medicinal substances.[53]

Where the single medicine protocol is ignored, and the prescription combines several different medicines and potencies, patient progress assessment is riddled with confusion. It is impossible to accurately judge with certainty many factors, including: which medicine in which potency induced a response; which medicine and potency produced a curative rather than non-curative response; which medicine is still affecting the vital force and which medicine isn't; which medicine and potency induced the vital force to overreact; which remedy and dose should be repeated and why. This 'throw everything at the kitchen sink' prescribing methodology is certainly much easier, but it risks exposing patients to avoidable uncontrollable extra suffering. It is the exact opposite of how Hahnemann intended homœopathy should be used.

The proper dose of homœopathic medicine is always a single substance in the smallest, single dose, given as infrequently as possible and only when patient response indicates repetition. The biggest incentive to adhere to this rule, is this:

The well informed and conscientiously careful physician will never be in a position to require an antidote in his practice if he will begin, as he should, to give the selected medicine in the smallest possible dose.[54]

Hahnemann's reasoning for always administering the single substance is as follows:

As the true physician finds in simple medicines, administered single and uncombined, all that he can possibly desire (artificial disease-forces which are able by homœopathic power completely to overpower, extinguish, and

---

[53] Dr. S. Hahnemann, *The Organon of Medicine*, §273

[54] Ibid §249 F/n 136

permanently cure natural diseases), he will, mindful of the wise maxim that 'it is wrong to attempt to employ complex means when simple means suffice,' never think of giving as a remedy any but a single, simple medicinal substance; for these reasons also, because even though the simple medicines were thoroughly proved with respect to their peculiar effects on the unimpaired healthy state of man, it is yet impossible to foresee how two and more medicinal substances might, when compounded, hinder and alter each other's actions on the human body; and because on the other hand, a simple medicinal substance when used in diseases, the totality of whose symptoms is accurately known, renders efficient air by itself alone, if it be homœopathically selected.[55]

Pure homœopathic healing artists never give a medicine without scheduling a progress report appointment. The illness is in motion, the vital force is in constant motion, and there are shifts in bodily functions. Practitioners have a duty to diligently monitor patient responses at certain intervals depending on whether the potency prescribed is centesimal or LM/Q and the state of illness is chronic or acute, for evidence of a directional shift of symptoms, to evaluate whether the vital force is responding curatively or not. Patients must never be left on the wrong medicine for too long. It invites serious avoidable harm.

Which brings us to the last fixed fundamental principle.

The natural direction of cure

To understand this principle correctly, the practitioner must be aware of what happens once the homœopathically selected medicine has been absorbed into the body and the vital force responds.

Before the medicine is taken, during the long struggle to regain balance, the weakened vital force becomes more and more, as it were, distracted and confused about how to free itself from harm. It sends out numerous distress signals. When it receives a correct dose of the correctly selected homœopathic medicine—a simulated, similar, but slightly magnified version of the illness, which is strong enough to grab

[55] Ibid §274

the full attention of the vital force but not overwhelm it—clarity replaces confusion. The power of medicine and the prevailing power of vital force unite. The vital force is compelled to increase its strength by degrees. At last its strength increases to the point where it becomes more far more powerful than the original natural illness and eventually overpowers the medicinally artificial simulated illness, order replaces chaos and equilibrium is restored throughout the body. As soon as the practitioner sees the quality of health restored, dosing stops and the apparent increase of the disease caused by the homœopathic medicine disappears by itself. The vital force reigns supreme over its domain. Life goes on.[56]

In correct homœopathic treatment of a chronic illness that has been left alone and not irritated by medical mismanagement of any kind, a curative response is understood to take place when the patient's strength increases right from the start and continues to improve. This is followed by mental and emotional improvement, followed by relief from discomfort in the outer physical parts of the body. This inward—outwards directional shift indicates that order is gradually being restored throughout the body.[57] All is well when diseases go from centre to circumference, out from the centres of life, out from the heart lungs, brain and spine, out from the interior to the extremities.[58] The innermost vital organs under greatest threat, tend to heal first, less vital organs recover later. For some patients, symptoms simultaneously disappear in a north-to-south direction—from head to hands and feet.[59]

It is imperative to understand that illnesses that have been irritated —complicated by prior medical mismanagement of some kind—tend to heal much more slowly. The road to recovery is full of twists, turns

---

[56] Dr. S. Hahnemann, *The Organon of Medicine*, Author's Preface to the Sixth edition, and §29, and *The Chronic Diseases: Their Peculiar Nature and their Homœopathic Cure*; Preface to the Fourth Volume.

[57] Dr. S. Hahnemann, *Chronic Diseases: Their Peculiar Nature and Their Homœopathic Cure*

[58] Dr. J. T. Kent, *Lectures on Homœopathic Philosophy*,

[59] Dr. H. A. Roberts, *The Principles and Art of Cure by Homœopathy*

and detours. Even so the curative direction of such illness is still always inwards–outward, and never outwards–inward.

A simple example of the direction of cure is an individual who suffers mental depression and skin symptoms. After treatment, the mental depression lifts first. Later on the skin symptoms improve, or disappear. Were the skin condition to recover first without improvement of the depression, or the depression worsen while the skin improves, that response indicates the patient is moving in the non-curative wrong direction. Symptoms that move outwards–inward, from skin to mind or brain, from less vital organ to more vital organ (e.g. in the case of rheumatic fever, if the joints get better first and heart condition worsens) indicate that the illness has been strengthened and continues unabated. The influence of the medicine on the vital force must be interrupted immediately and appropriate non-medicinal adjunctive measures implemented. The case needs to be urgently restudied and if necessary a different medicine selected, one that shares greater symptom-similarity with the illness, or where the same remedy is indicated, careful consideration be given to changing from 'c' to LM/Q potency to minimise a possible over reaction.

Those nine fixed fundamental principles: *Vital force of nature; Inherent predispositions to illness; Susceptibility: action and reaction; Totality of characteristic individualising symptoms; Dilution potentiation and the infinitesimal dose; Know the curative power of each individual medicine; Let likes be cured with likes—Similia Similibus Curentur; Proper dose: single substance, single dose, and Natural direction of cure*, define and identify homœopathy for all time.

> Thus homœopathy is a perfectly simple system of medicine, remaining always fixed in its principles as in its practice, which like the doctrine whereon is based, if rightly apprehended, will be found to be complete (and therefore serviceable). What is clearly pure in doctrine and practice should be self-evident, and all backward sliding to the pernicious routinism of the old school that is as much its antithesis as night is to day, should cease to vaunt itself with the honorable name name of Homœopathy.[60]

---

[60] Dr. S. Hahnemann, *The Organon of Medicine*, Sixth Final Edition, Author's Preface

2

Health Disease and Cure

This topic was touched on in the last chapter. However, let's take a deeper look.

In homœopathy, health is where the progress of life continues unimpeded. The life principle, vital force of nature at the core of our being is free flowing and powerful enough to maintain all regions of the mind and body in harmony and order so that we may achieve our full potential. Without medicine of any kind, the vital force is sufficient to correct minor imbalances with little or no disruption. Our susceptibility and reaction to harmful influences is proportionate and appropriate. We recover quickly.

Illness reflects the degree to which the progress of life is impeded and we are unable to fulfil our full potential. Our susceptibility to harmful influences is disproportionate. Regularity of life is disturbed at the core of our being and ripples outwards until it is expressed by symptoms and irregularities. The severity and region of discomfort indicate how far towards the core a harmful influence has penetrated and how much strength still prevails in the vital force. Where the vital force of nature is sufficient, the struggle will be strong, effective and short. Where the vital force is insufficient, the struggle will be weak, prolonged, chaotic, intermittent or ineffective, it will strive to save life no matter what this entails, often with the largest sacrifices or destruction of life itself.[61]

Cure using homœopathy removes signs, symptoms and uncomfortable sensations produced *naturally* during illness by harnessing the body's innate curative process, which is understood to be already underway but has stalled. The medicine taken nudges the vital force in the right direction to resume and finish the job it started.

In homœopathic practice, symptoms serve many very useful purposes. Each person's unique state of disorder manifests in patterns of symptoms peculiar to that individual. Those symptoms are the single infallible guide to selecting the most symptom-similar homœopathic medicine. Strangely, the more bothersome a symptom is, or the more symptoms there are, the more likely sufficient strength of vital force still prevails in the patient to bring about recovery, because it is still trying different ways to free itself from harm. Fewer bothersome symptoms experienced by an extremely unwell patient indicate the vital force is unable to keep trying to rid itself of harm, which makes finding a suitable symptom-similar remedy less likely. It's *the original natural illness symptom totality picture alone* that directs the practitioner to the most suitable symptom-similar medicine. Curability depends on a homœopathic practitioner's understanding of which symptoms should be treated and which should not. Symptoms accidentally, unconsciously or deliberately induced by patients' lifestyles should not be confused with signs of chronic disease. Provided no chronic predisposition to illness lurks in the body, those symptoms tend to disappear in response to appropriate patient education, or when living conditions improve.[62]

Often we forget how easy it is to stay healthy without medicine. Patient or guardian education about reasonable lifestyle adjustments to assist the vital force and enhance recovery is an essential part of homœopathic practice.

The potential for recovery using homœopathy requires several things to occur: the ability of a particular body to produce symptoms and clearly signal its distress; the patient or guardian's ability to observe and

---

[61] Dr. S. Hahnemann, *The Organon of Medicine*, Sixth edition, §22 F/n 12

[62] Ibid §77

describe those uncomfortable sensations and the practitioner's ability to make the perfect medicine and dose selection that will encourage the patient's vital force to remove the symptoms. In homœopathy the curative power of a symptom-similar medicine depends on a) the degree of similarity between the symptoms it causes when taken by healthy people and the symptoms experienced by each patient, and b) the strength of the medicinal dose selected and administered, which must be slightly stronger than the prevailing strength of the vital force.

Once the medicine is absorbed through the sentient nerves into the organism, the vital force is presented with a magnified and intensified artificial version of the original natural disorder and instinctively reacts against it. Gradually the power of the vital force increases to such a degree that it becomes far more powerful than both the artificial symptoms produced by the homœopathic medicine, which simulates the disease, and the symptoms of original natural disease itself. The disease yields to the overwhelming power of the individual's newly invigorated vital force. The symptoms soon lose their power, disappear by themselves and leave the patient free from disease. Thus liberated, the vital force gently restores harmony throughout the whole spiritual, mental, emotional and physical organism, and continues to carry life on in health. Recovery will be certain in proportion to the strength with which the vital force prevails in the patient.[63] In accordance with the natural direction of cure, symptoms that appeared most recently tend to disappear first, those that appeared a long time ago would disappear later. That said, very complicated illness often takes a less orderly route.

Once the individual's innate self-recovery power is strengthened and reestablished, susceptibility to sickness is decreased, freeing that person to fulfil their full potential in life.

However, Hahnemann never claimed homœopathy to be a cure-all. Like all medical systems, it has its limitations, which he honestly acknowledged.[64] It is wise to be realistic about expectations for

---

[63] Dr. S. Hahnemann, *The Organon of Medicine*, Author's Preface to the Sixth edition, and §29, and *The Chronic Diseases: Their Peculiar Nature and Their Homœopathic Cure*, Preface to the Fourth Volume.

[64] Dr. S. Hahnemann, *The Organon of Medicine*, Sixth edition, §74, §75

complete and smooth recovery, especially where there's a history of mainstream and homœopathic medical systems used concurrently or alternately.

Hahnemann's experiments with homœopathic medicines and healthy people proved all medicines have the power to affect us always, unconditionally. That being true, individuals whose prior treatment includes multiple large physiological dose drugs, or ill-chosen homœopathic medicines for extended periods of time, may suffer lasting side effect symptoms of those medicines alongside symptoms of the original natural illness, which distort the portrait of the original natural illness. He says that:

> Much more frequent than the natural diseases associating with complicating one another in the same body are the morbid complications which the inappropriate medical treatment (the allopathic[65] method) is apt to produce by the long-continued employment of unsuitable drugs. To the natural disease, which it is proposed to cure, there are then added, by the constant repetition of the unsuitable medicinal agent, the new, often very tedious, morbid conditions corresponding to the nature of this agent; these gradually coalesce with and complicate the chronic malady which is dissimilar to them (which they were unable to cure by similarity of action, that is, homœopathically), adding to the old disease, a new dissimilar, artificial malady of a chronic nature, an thus give the patient a double in place of a single disease, that is to say, render him much worse and more difficult to cure, often quite incurable.[66]

> These inroads on human health effected by the allopathic non-healing art (more particularly in recent times) are of all chronic illnesses, the most deplorable, the most incurable; and I regret to add that it is apparently impossible to discover or hit upon any remedies for their cure when they have reached any considerable height.[67]

Unnatural side-effect symptoms may only disappear when the medicine that caused them is stopped, and that only happens where the

---

[65] Medical practice that aims to combat disease by administering remedies that produce effects different from and opposite to those produced by the disease experienced. The term 'Allopathy, allopathic' is from the Greek, alloison pathos, meaning 'heterogeneous', or 'unlike' disease.

[66] Dr. S. Hahnemann, *The Organon of Medicine,* Sixth edition, §41

[67] Ibid §75

prescribing physician deems it safe to do so. With the vital force having been burdened for a long time, drug reduction is the equivalent of taking the lid off a pressure cooker before it is safe to do so. All hell may break loose. It's extremely dangerous to encourage anyone to stop any medications without physician consent to a very slow and gentle, graduated drug reduction protocol carefully monitored by the prescribing physician. Depending how strong the medicines are, which organs are affected and always provided there is enough strength left in the patient to withstand the discomfort, it may take years for all those unnatural side-effect symptoms to disappear. Where sufficient vital force strength prevails and homœopathy is used proficiently, sometimes the original *natural* symptoms re-emerge in an intensified version of how they first appeared before medicines masked them. They may be clearer, but the suffering is often terrible. The natural symptoms may eventually subside, but medicinal side-effect symptoms may still remain. Sometimes the vital force has been so severely constrained and doubly disturbed by prior medicinal and surgical treatment that it founders. If the vital force is to be helped back on track, rigorous practitioner adherence to all the fixed fundamental principles of homœopathy is essential. The obstacles to recovery are immense, with the process being akin to unravelling a Gordian knot. For homœopathy to be effective, it is crucial that the artificially induced, unnatural side effect symptoms of medicines are identified and excluded from the homœopathic prescription basis which must always reflect the original portrait of the illness prior to medical treatment.

There are two ways to do this. First, look up the mainstream medicines taken in an online database such as www.drugs.com and check the list of side effects against those reported in the patient examination. Second, review the timeline of patient illness progress. Typically, after one condition received prior unsuitable treatment, another condition emerged. This raises doubts about the natural occurrence of that second condition. Where there's doubt, chuck it out!

To avoid overwhelming an already severely weakened vital force, selection and administration of homœopathic medicines in optimal minimal doses and at proper intervals between doses must be undertaken judiciously. As mentioned earlier, improper use of homœopathic medicines, those selected and administered for groups of symptoms rather than the totality of symptoms, causes more harm than good, as it tends to rivet the constitutional state upon the patient and make him incurable.[68]

In many countries, homœopathic treatment is an out-of-pocket expense. Knowing what hard earned cash will buy is important. How rapidly we may recover from chronic illness using homœopathy depends on other factors:

The individual's age; the number of years the individual has suffered illness; whether the individual has been medically mismanaged by an excess of allopathic treatments, or as often happens mismanaged into incurableness; how much, self-healing vital force remains; the suitability of the homœopathic remedy dose and intervals between doses the practitioner selected.

Only an ordinary ignorant practitioner can lightly promise to cure a severe inveterate disease in four to six weeks. The nature of the case forbids hastening the cure.

The cure of great chronic diseases of ten, twenty, thirty and more years' standing, (if they have not been mismanaged by an excess of allopathic treatment, or indeed, as is often the case, mismanaged into incurableness) may be said to be quickly annihilated if this is achieved in one or two years. If with younger, robust persons this takes place in one-half the time, then on the other hand in advanced age, even with the best treatment on the part of the physician and the most punctual observance of rules on the part of the patient and his attendants, considerable time must be added to the usual period of the cure. It will also be found intelligible that such a long-continued (psoric) chronic disease, the original [inherited predisposition] miasm of which has had so much time and opportunity in a long life to insert its parasitical roots as it were, into all the joints of the tender edifice of life, is at last so intimately interwoven with the organism that even with the most appropriate medical treatment, careful mode of life and observances of the rules on the part of the patient, great patience and sufficient time will be required to destroy this many armed polypus in all its parts, while sparing the independence of the organism [the body] and its powers.[69]

---

[68] Dr. J. T. Kent, *Lectures on Homœopathic Philosophy*

[69] Dr. S. Hahnemann, *The Chronic Diseases: Their Peculiar Nature and Their Homœopathic Cure.*

Even though complete health restoration takes time, the strength of young or old patients ought to continually increase from the start of the correct treatment.[70]

When using homœopathy, an individual's potential for recovery is hindered by:

- Practitioner lack of knowledge proficiency and due diligence in pure method homœopathic practice.
- Prolonged prior administration of ineffective medication often repeated in rapid succession in increasingly stronger doses.
- Prior administration of more than one known substance combined in one homœopathic prescription that induced new and often ineradicable medicinal illnesses.[71]
- Continuing unavoidable concurrent use of strong single or combined psychotropic, hypnotic, narcotic or sedative, etc., medicines.
- Overmedication, inducing an unnatural oversensitive vital force that overreacts to all medicines.
- Patients violating the rules for recovery, e.g. concurrent self-medicating homœopathic medicine without practitioner knowledge or consent.
- Administration of medicinal doses that are too strong.
- Improper intervals between doses of homœopathic medicines.
- Administration of a remedy improperly based on one or two symptoms versus properly selecting a symptom-similar medicine that fits the totality of characteristic, individualising symptoms.
- Improper selection and administration of homœopathic remedies based on the end *results* of illness alone, versus the *origins and results* of illness.
- A practitioner fails to elicit individualising features of illness.

---

[70] Dr. S. Hahnemann, *The Chronic Diseases: Their Peculiar Nature and Their Homœopathic Cure.*

[71] Dr. S. Hahnemann, *The Organon of Medicine*, Sixth edition, Author's Preface, §41, §74 – §76, §274

- There are few or no symptoms.
- The patient forgets, or for some reason conceals, symptoms from the practitioner.
- Results of disease have produced irreparable tissue destruction and the patient experiences severe weakness. [72]

Potential for recovery is increased when the practitioner thoroughly understands the significance of what is observed, sees through the patient's suffering to the centre of the disorder and the beleaguered vital force, and knows how to secure rapid, gentle and continuous health proficiently.

---

[72] *Kent's, New Remedies, Clinical Cases, Lesser Writings, Aphorisms & Precepts,* compiled by Dr. W.W. Sherwood. Article: The Second Prescription

3

Knowledge of the Disease or, The Patient Examination

This chapter describes the effective homœopathic patient examination which provides knowledge about the disease and what is to be cured. This is where true practitioners of homœopathy put the first four fixed principles of homœopathic practice through their paces. A minimal dose of the author's clinical experience is included to enhance clarity.

In authentic homœopathic practice, health restoration is never conducted according to a one-size-fits-all, predetermined, preconceived, generalised plan for treatment of a specific named disease. To the frequently asked question what's the best homœopathic remedy for depression, asthma, rheumatism, diarrhoea, diabetes, hypothyroidism, etc., the correct homœopathic answer is always: the one indicated by the particular uncomfortable symptoms experienced by each patient. That is why studies designed to test the effectiveness of homœopathy by applying the predetermined prescribing method used in ordinary medical practice, to provide the public with information about what specific homœopathic medicine should be administered to relieve which specific symptoms or diseases, are misguided. They demonstrate not only the study designer's profound misunderstanding of the true purpose of homœopathy and its legitimate sphere of operation, but also denial of the truth that the homœopathic and allopathic medical systems are exact opposites that cannot approach each other or unite. Anyone who thinks they can does not understand either system of medicine.[73] Routine prescribing is antithetical to homœopathy as night is to day. Therefore, it is questionable whether or not the results of such studies provides the public with evidence of the effectiveness or ineffectiveness of homœopathy.

In homœopathy, each patient and their disease is understood to be completely different from all other similar states of suffering. Therefore a medicine and dose prescribed for one patient and their symptoms will differ from that selected for someone else experiencing similar symptoms.

This is best illustrated when two people discuss their headaches in detail. Even though the discomfort experienced by both is in same region of the body, their exact experience of it is different. For example, the exact location, causation, type and intensity of pain or other sensations that might be felt in unrelated regions of the body at the same time as the headache will be completely different. Factors that make one person feel better or worse will differ from factors that affect the other person. In homœopathy, it's the totality of those minor and major differences between their suffering that guides practitioners to the symptom-similar medicine and dose for each person's headache. And, depending on exactly how each one responds, intervals between each dose will be different.'

For most people, falling ill is frightening. What does the discomfort mean? What's going to happen? Although we want to find out what the matter is, the mere thought of undergoing a formal patient examination is extremely worrying. The typical mainstream medical consultation is a fifteen-minute, test-driven, poking and prodding, maybe strip naked whirlwind.

Mercifully, the homœopathic patient examination is completely different. When conducted by an expert practitioner it's a gentle process, more like sitting for a portrait painter, except you're allowed to

---

[73] Dr. S. Hahnemann, *The Organon of Medicine*, Sixth edition, §52

move around! For practitioners to get a deep sense of who each person is and understand exactly how they are affected by their symptoms, it is wise to schedule an unrestricted amount of time, so that the patient only needs to bare their soul once, rather than several times in short succession. To trace a complete, multidimensional, faithful, image of each person and their unique experience of suffering, the practitioner listens extremely attentively to the story of the illness and notes down the exact descriptions of each symptom or condition. Proficiency depends on the acuteness of intellectual, sensory and observational faculties of the practitioner. The paintbrush and canvas are the pen and paper, the exact words used by each patient to describe everything about their suffering is the palette.

The most discreet, least disruptive homœopathic case-taking method, and the one used for all treatment phases, is one that is written down word-for-word. A verbatim record of the interview eliminates relying on practitioner memory and avoids the potential for the practitioner to confuse the symptoms of one patient with those of another. However, those unskilled in the verbatim reporting technique, and others tend to document consultations using computers and audiovisual technology. Although this method might be convenient in the short term, it is wise to consider it a double-edged sword as it could create a serious psychological barrier, similar to putting a desk between patient and practitioner. The typing noise might distract and irritate some sensitive people. Others, especially elders, not wishing to appear uncooperative might agree to computer use, but may view its presence as a significant deterrent to disclosing certain extremely useful but private information. The practitioner's duty includes not only *listening,* but also *observing* patients as they describe their illness history. A particular gesture or facial expression in response to a question might offer a completely new and beneficial line of inquiry. Constantly glancing at a computer screen or looking down at the keyboard while typing, insinuates indifference and risks missing a potentially significant opportunity for deeper investigation. Anticipating equipment failure risks interrupting practitioner concentration, actual failure of technology will distract any patient. What might have been important clues to solve the puzzle are lost forever. Then there is the double time needed to view the video to make sure you didn't miss anything.

The effective patient examination not only puts patients at ease, it also puts patient comfort over practitioner convenience.

One time, before I could show them where to sit, my new patient strode in and sat down in what I regard as my seat. Turning on a sixpence, I grabbed pen and pad and settled into what I considered to be the patient's seat.

Then there was the mid-winter consultation I almost froze to death. The patient requested that all windows be opened and no heating to be in the room. Lesson learned, always wear layers for consultations.

Before many secrets, long-hidden thoughts or emotions that are far too difficult or too painful to divulge to a complete stranger may be revealed, patient–practitioner trust and confidence must be built. The practitioner is like an archaeologist, brushing away centuries of dust to reveal a precious artifact.

At the end of a well-taken history, a detailed map of the exact route taken by the vital force as it struggles to escape from harmful influences must emerge. This map leads directly to the start of that struggle, the root of the turmoil, the reason that individual has become sick in that particular way at that particular time in their life. Tracing the complete, true image of the illness requires us to understand everything that was going on at the beginning of the illness during its earliest manifestations, and everything that happened along the path as the illness progressed. It means tracking back through a chronology of events, symptoms and conditions to the original form of the illness, before it was changed and masked by different treatments.

The proper homœopathic patient examination invites the stricken vital force to display and release its distress so that the practitioner accurately understands and captures on paper everything about each patient and their symptoms. It scrutinises everything and discovers all the general and particular individualising features that identify and portray the unique symptom image totality of suffering. It means perceiving patterns and grasping hold of the thread that links everything together, that leads patient and practitioner through a labyrinth to the central suffering.

The goal of the examination is to free the patient's vital force from the burden of symptoms, and allow the individual to feel as comfortable about discussing their illness as they would be describing it to a trusted friend.

The best way to achieve that objective is for the practitioner to create a tranquil environment. Mobile phones should be turned off, answer machines silenced and message lights covered up. The room is best arranged in such a way that patient and practitioner sit square on, not too far away from or too close to each other, with one small table at the side of each person for the necessary accoutrements.

To make the patient forget that she or he is being examined, expert practitioners strive for invisibility. They temporarily eschew personal religious insignia and wear muted rather than vibrant colours. They invite patients to understand for themselves why they have fallen ill and to discover ways in which they may avoid falling ill in the future. The best examinations are those where the healing process leaps forward. The worst ones are those where the consult ends and the practitioner is left with tens of pages of vague descriptions of symptoms without individualising characteristic features, and insufficient information for a curative prescription to be made. Selecting a medicine based on a paucity of information will be likely to aggravate illness rather than cure it.

The proficient practitioner adjusts swiftly to each patient's personality, assumes an open, inviting posture, and exhibits a demeanour that is:

- Calm
- Dignified
- Quiet
- Empathetic
- Confident
- Simple and direct
- Without self-importance
- Business-like, but not too formal
- Cheerful, but not flippant
- Serious, but not grave or funereal

- Painstaking and systematic

To obtain the highest quality information, practitioners:

- Observe objective phenomena accurately and discretely, although without seeming to do so.
- Record statements quietly without attracting notice.
- Do not laugh at or correct patient errors.
- Do not hurry the patient.

In Hahnemann's pure homœopathy, practitioners are required to summon a particular state of mind: to be the unprejudiced observer where we leave our own suffering, personal likes and dislikes, value systems as well as speculations, preconceptions about patients and different homœopathic remedies outside the consulting room and far away from the case at hand. Instead of speculating and hypothesising about the cause and nature of each individual's illness, we:

...Direct all our thoughts upon the matter we have in hand, come out of ourselves, as it were, and fasten ourselves, so to speak, on it, so that nothing that is truly present that has to do with the subject, and that can be ascertained by all the senses, may escape us.

For the time being, poetic fancy, fantastic wit and speculation must be suspended and all overstrained reasoning, forced interpretation and tendency to explain away things must be suppressed. The duty of the observer is only to take notice of the phenomena and their course; his attention should be on the watch, not only that nothing truly present escape his attention, but that also what he observes be understood exactly as it is.[74]

Stepping out of ourselves frees us to wholeheartedly focus on someone else's struggle, we must exert the will and intellect to concentrate on creating a sanctuary, a confidential healing atmosphere in which the patient is put at ease and able to speak freely without shame or fear of being judged about sexual functions, menstrual flow, their private innermost thoughts and feelings (their loves, hates, desires, aversions, views, values), and anything else that affects them and makes them feel ill.

---

[74]Dr. S. Hahnemann, *Materia Medica Pura,*

Accustomed to mainstream medical practice tell all in five minutes or less protocols, the story of the illness tends to tumble out at breakneck speed. It centres on current troubles rather than how it all started. A gentle nudge is needed to complete the whole story.

At the beginning of the examination, advise the patient to speak slowly so that you may accurately take down in writing the important parts of what the patient says in the exact expressions used.[75]

The homœopathic patient examination draws a recognisable portrait of the illness in its totality. Every disease has its symptom mug-shot likeness stored in the homœopathic medicine information database. The task is to find that medicine. To do that we need to elicit individualising symptoms in these categories:

- Striking, Singular, Uncommon and Peculiar (characteristic) symptoms
- General Mental, Emotional Disposition and modifying features
- Sleep disturbances and modifying features
- General Physical Disposition and modifying features
- Particulars: region, affinity, location, extensions, sensations and modifying features
- Sensations and modifying features

To create a true homœopathic, multidimensional likeness of each patient's illness requires gathering information not only about the symptoms suffered throughout the course of the illness, but also about their lifestyle and quality of mind, soul and body. All the most striking, singular, uncommon and peculiar characteristic symptoms must be investigated, elicited and documented. To individualise an illness, practitioners apply a particular intellectual perspective: one that discriminates between symptoms produced by the natural illness and the side-effect symptoms from medicines; one that views an illness from its beginning through to its end and back again; from its centre to its circumference, innermost to outermost. Hahnemann teaches that

---

[75] Dr. S. Hahnemann, *The Organon of Medicine*, Sixth edition, §84

the proper homœopathic patient examination investigates the whole state of the patient. This includes the internal causes as far as they are remembered, and the causes of continuing illness.

To unlock the door to the truth about each illness, practitioners of homœopathy in the true sense of the word are:

> Unprejudiced, indefatigable, discriminating, perceptive, persevering, and possesses that quality of great patience, supported by the power of the will, penetrating intellect, and reflective reasoning, which is not usually met with among ordinary physicians even in a moderate degree. Unfettered judgment, all over powers of concentration, the capacity and habit of noticing carefully, correctly; the capability of refining the perceptions of the senses; at the same time preserve the necessary coolness, calmness, and firmness of judgment together with a constant distrust of our own powers of apprehension. The art of drawing from nature is also useful, as it enables us to attain directness in thinking and feeling, as well as appropriateness and simplicity in expressing our sensations. It also sharpens and practices our eye and thereby also our other senses, teaching us to form a true conception of objects, and to represent what we observe, truly and purely without any addition from fancy.[76]

Add to that list of prerequisites, the capacity to shift swiftly between lines of inquiry. It's a very tall order.

The most effective practitioners never ask leading questions that suggest the answer. Such suggestions seduce patients into giving a false answer and a false account of their symptoms. The practitioner always follows where the patient leads and goes at the patient's pace. As the story moves from one topic and symptom to another, Hahnemann advises the easiest way to get it all down accurately is to record each new circumstance and symptom on a separate line. To ensure enough space, it is wise to leave at least six lines space between each one, so that when the patient finishes the story, you can go back through the case filling in the gaps. Dates that things happened are marked in the left-hand margin. Traits of inherent predispositions to illness are marked in the right margin. Anything that is emphasised by gesture, voice pitch, or facial expression or appears unusual, prominent or

---

[76] Dr. S. Hahnemann, *Materia Medica Pura*,

troublesome is always underlined. That way, when reviewing the report before analysing the information, it's easily identified.

Minimum information about each symptom and condition should, where possible, include:

When it occurred for the first time

How it felt then

When and **how** it has changed

Time it occurs; e.g., morning, before noon, afternoon, evening, night, before or after midnight, monthly, seasonal, annually, etc.

Causations: the circumstance or condition that brought it on.

Locations: e.g., on the head, the forehead, the temples, sides, top, and back of the head; whether on the right or left side or whole of the head; whether it extends from one location to another.

Sensations: How the part feels, e.g. the kind of pain, burning, aching, sore, throbbing, etc.

Modifying factors: e.g., circumstances; conditions that make each aspect of suffering better or worse such as rest, motion, lying down, sitting, standing, walking, running, riding on horseback or in a vehicle, etc. Also, warmth or cold, open air or closed room, various pleasures, touch, exposure of the affected region, overheating, eating and drinking, emotions, dry or wet or stormy weather, sunlight or artificial light, etc. Anything the patient considers weird or strange about each symptom. The aim is to individualise the person and the disease, so anything and everything that makes us hesitate or meditate is useful.

If you understand exactly what constitutes the important parts of the story, and the intellectual faculty is firing on all cylinders it will automatically prompt you to record vital information. Here's an example:

I'm at the bedside. The patient has a high fever, is coughing up blood-streaked mucous, experiencing chest pains, wildly fluctuating respiration and heart rates, as in often observed in the illness known as 'pneumonia.' Those symptoms are all valuable.

However, to differentiate that person's experience of 'pneumonia' from everyone else's and find the most suitable homœopathic remedy for that person's particular version of pneumonia, I must elicit individualising features of the suffering. To do this, I encourage the patient by saying 'describe everything you possibly can about how you are feeling. I am interested in everything, every crumb, morsel of information, even if you think it's not important.'

The following individualising information comes out: 'It all came on after I got very chilled in a downpour without a jacket, and by the way, it's the weirdest thing, but everything is much worse after midnight—the pain, the coughing, everything. I know the time because I wake up and look at the clock. I have so much pain in my body, so I move about, even though when I begin to move, the pain is so much worse; but if I keep moving around, it gets better. That's why I go from the bed to the chair and back again and move around in the bed. I just can't lie or sit still. If I do, I get very anxious. By the way, the pains move around from one part of me to another. I never know where they are going to be next. The other thing is I just want to be by myself. That's strange because normally I love people around me. I can't get enough of them.' While the patient speaks, I observe a bright red triangular area at the tip of the tongue, the eyes are only partly open, the arms are drawn up to the chest, and the face is deathly pale with beads of perspiration on the chin. An odour of rotting flesh exudes from the mouth.

To be on the safe side and ensure nothing of significance escapes scrutiny, everything in the story—both common symptoms of the condition and the individualising features—must be noted down. The chronology of significant events and the illness, everything observed, experienced and stated by patients, constitute crucial parts of the story.

Look, listen and learn. Everything about homœopathic practice requires doing several things at the same time.

To look means to observe with the eyes while keeping them directed; to direct the attention; to consider; to examine; to await the appearance of anything; to take notice.

To listen means to hear with thoughtful attention and requires concentration.

To learn means to gain knowledge; to ascertain information by inquiry, study or investigation; to fix in the mind; to acquire understanding of or skill in an area of knowledge.

The face is an important communication tool. It is often said the heart is in the face. What a person experiences in their soul, is outwardly reflected in their facial expression. Therefore, it is very useful to observe patient facial expressions on arrival and departure, when the face is communicating and when it is at rest.

Expressions that can be seen on faces include: astonishment, infatuation, intoxication, bewilderment, confusion, distress, fierceness, foolishness, fright, haggardness, happiness, idiocy, old-looking, pinched, sickly, sleepy, stupid, sullenness, fatigue, vacant, wildness, worry and many other feelings. The sensation and degree of pain is often reflected in facial expressions.

There are many mental and emotional characteristics to be observed without the patient saying a word. These include: fear, shock, shyness, whether they are easily hurt, angered, irritated, startled, embarrassment, exhilaration, haughtiness, recklessness, suspicion, laughter, memory weakness, sighing, tendency to be quiet or restless or tearful when talking about certain symptoms or topics, among others.

In homœopathic practice, it is inappropriate for practitioners to express emotions in response to anything the patient-guardian says. If the history provokes anger or weeping, you must relax. It will soon pass. Bear witness rather than become afraid or rush to comfort. Hold your own emotions in check. Some patients are deeply disturbed by a practitioner showing emotion. They discontinue telling their story. Practitioner and patient become seriously distracted. The therapeutic role reverses and the cared-for becomes the caregiver. Practitioner concentration is interrupted, which severely reduces the practitioner's ability to understand exactly what the patient is saying. The most important piece of information to guide the practitioner to the correct remedy could be lost forever.

A case well-taken is a case half-cured. A well-conducted patient examination provides enough time for the story of the illness to be told at a leisurely pace and in its entirety. It is essential that practitioners do not judge or reach conclusions about the person or the illness without first hearing the whole history or completing a full examination. To be effective, the practitioner's observations and inquiries are independent and neutral; the mind is held in that unprejudiced state, *tabula rasa*. It is a blank slate waiting to be freshly written upon by each patient. Suspension of prejudice is the most essential and the most difficult practitioner skill required in patient examinations. It requires great humility and the ability to examine the conscience to identify all discriminatory tendencies.

To suspend prejudice requires being aware of it, acknowledging it, taking responsibility for it, and then controlling the inappropriate impulse to be judgemental. That takes practitioner intelligence, courage and extraordinary strength of will and character. Unfettered by prejudice of any kind, we experience freedom to wholeheartedly bear witness to the patient's suffering with greater compassion and clarity, and we are better placed to help restore health. Prejudice takes many forms.

Prejudice, bias against or towards certain remedies, is to be avoided.[77]

One of the most important things is to keep out of the mind, in an examination of the case, some other case that has appeared to be similar. If this is not done, the mind will be prejudiced in spite of your best endeavors. I have to fight that with every fresh case I come to. I have to labor to keep myself from thinking about things I have cured like that before, because it would prejudice my mind.

The purpose of all this is that you will go away and examine the patient with an unprejudiced mind, that you will consider only the case before you, that you will have nothing in mind that will distract your attention, that you may not think of things that preceded it and find out from among them a remedy while examining the patient. If you are biased in your judgment and examine the patient towards a certain remedy, in many instances this will prove to be fatal. Have no remedy in mind until you have everything that you can get on paper. Have it all written down carefully then, if upon examining it in relation to remedies, you are unable to distinguish between three or four remedies, you can go back and re-examine the patient with reference to those three or four remedies.

---

[77] Dr. S. Hahnemann, *The Organon of Medicine*, Sixth edition, §257

That is the only possible time you try to fit a remedy, or image of a remedy, while examining a patient. Get all the symptoms first and then commence your analysis in relation to remedies.[78]

Any one of hundreds medicines could be the one most suitable for a particular person with a particular illness.

This is exactly why the trend in homœopathic education to mimic ordinary medical training—to rote learn, to memorise certain small groups of keynote symptoms to brand a few remedies on the brain—is so damaging to homœopathy. It encourages backsliding to old school routinism. During such an examination, there is a very strong potential for those particular remedies to flood and bias the practitioner's mind. Before the case is heard in its entirety, the practitioner reaches a conclusion about the suitability of a particular remedy. For example, where the practitioner observes red lips, the memory suggests the probability of Sulphur. Rote learned keynote symptoms creep in. The practitioner asks the patient questions to confirm the idea of Sulphur such as: Do you feel a sensation of emptiness before noon? How do you feel standing for a while? Do you put your feet out of the bed at night because they are burning? You probably drink a lot and don't eat much, right?

In that line of questioning, using closed, leading questions rather than properly listening to and using the patient's volunteered symptom descriptions as the only true indicator of the most suitable remedy, the practitioner improperly directs the patient towards offering information about a specific remedy which the practitioner has predetermined the patient needs. Dr. Pierre Schmidt calls that the Torpedo Inquiry method, suggesting that the truth is torpedoed. He offers the following advice to eliminate this significant obstacle to cure:

When you are taking the case of a patient and you see it is Pulsatilla, you write in the corner of your case paper, Pulsatilla. Now, after ten minutes, it is typically Nux Vomica, so you put down Nux Vomica. Then you see symptoms of Arsenicum and you put down Arsenicum. At the end of the questioning, you have twenty different remedies because, of course, they are symptoms of these remedies that you remember. Therefore, your memory is

---

[78] Dr. J.T. Kent, *Lectures on Homœopathic Philosophy*

very good; but in spite of being good, you cannot know fifteen hundred pages of the Repertory (the index of symptoms experienced during the trials of each homœopathic remedy). When you put down the remedies on the side, the mind is free, neutral, and you can begin to study the case independently of any other case you have seen.[79]

There is so much more to examining a patient homœopathically than sitting down with the patient at the appointed time. The practitioner puts the private life on hold, ignites the homœopathic intellect, and focuses every cell in the body on the sick person and the illness.

Practitioners proficient in homœopathic patient examination adopt a relaxed, open, inviting, receptive and attending composure. They possess solid, highly developed senses and are prepared to traverse unknown territory. Ready to record everything that could lead, indirectly or directly, to the appropriate selection of the remedy with the greatest potential to cure the disease, they witness without judgement, observe and faithfully trace the portrait of each particular illness. Instead of jumping to conclusions and asking closed questions that invite Yes or No answers, they formulate and ask open questions, such as Why? How? When? Where? And prompt the patient to think deeply about their illness. My patients will tell you I'm always saying 'I am going to be silent a moment while I think how to ask my next question.' In these instances, often I am just about to ask my question, when the patient—having used the silence to think about something— comes out with an unexpected and brilliant gem of information. So, off we go down a valuable new line of inquiry. Just make sure you make a note of question you were going to ask before the gem dropped in your lap.

Formulating open questions

Not knowing exactly what territory is going to be covered by each patient examination makes framing open questions quickly, without

---

[79] Dr. P Schmidt, *The Art of Case Taking*

preparation difficult to do. It requires exceptional agility of practitioner intellect.

To give you some idea of how to formulate open questions, let's tackle the most challenging ones, those related to the mental and emotional disposition. Once you have understood how to ask those questions, you will find it easier to formulate open questions related to other areas.

Not in away intended to be an exhaustive list of mind-related open questions, but only to offer a few ideas regarding how such questions might be framed, the following suggestions might be worth considering. To ensure proper understanding of answers to these questions, never assume you know what is meant by the answer, always ask for examples.

- Describe your overall state of mind and any changes that affect you…give me an example.

- Describe your emotional state and any changes that affect you.

- Describe the things that are on your mind most of the time and may bother you.

- Tell me as much as you know or remember about your birth.

- Describe your childhood.

- Describe your adolescence.

- As far back as you can remember, describe all the significant changes you have experienced in your life.

- How do you get along with family members?

- Describe everything you love about life and your personality.

- Describe everything you hate about life and your personality.

- Tell me everything that delights you.

- Tell me all about your cravings, aversions, longings, yearnings.

- How do you experience and express emotion?

- Which emotions do you experience or express most of the time?

- How are you affected by emotions?

- Which emotions bother you?

- Why do they bother you?

- Over the years what changes have you experienced in your expression of emotions?

- Describe everything that has changed or makes you feel uncomfortable about your ability to:

    o Think

    o Understand

    o Concentrate

    o Remember

- For women: How is your mental emotional disposition affected before, during, of after menstruation?

In veterinary homœopathic practice animal expressions of emotions are carefully observed and examined. The wellbeing of animals is so intimately tied to their owner, observing animal-guardian interactions is essential for veterinarians treating pets. A useful veterinary open question for pet owners is: Describe aspects you love/hate about your pet's personality, and aspects that change when he is unwell.

Veterinarians serving farm animals need to be more creative in formulating their open questions and focus on using their observational skills extremely effectively, if they want to gain similar information.

It is essential to guide companion animal guardians *away from speculative anthropomorphic information* and towards evidential information. You are hoping for evidence of emotions like this:

- **Sounds:** purring, roaring, barking, growling, whimpering, bleating, screaming, singing, shrieking, spitting, hissing, clacking, neighing, humming, buzzing, rattling, bellowing.

- **Skin changes**: erect rigid bristling fur, feathers, or shedding. Erect ears, tails, wings, spines arms etc.

- **Gestures:** motion of body parts: wagging tails, open/closed mouth/beaks; chewing, biting; kicking; relaxed or stiff gait; pawing the ground; rubbing, licking own body parts. Sight directed forward; to the side; exposure of whites of eyes; dilated nostrils; lips drawn back, exposure of teeth; arching spine; inflation of whole or part of body; lying; voiding of urine or bowels.

- **Complete stillness:** of the body, in whole or in part to avoid pain or detection.

When considering alterations of health in animals, it is wise not to overlook the possible affect of the surgical removal of their healthy reproductive organs. It is important to know whether there were any marked behavioural or other changes that occurred since that surgery.

Whether human or animal the degree to which lack the freedom to live, feel, think and act as we want or to find meaning in life is the degree to which we become ill.

In human homœopathic practice basing remedy selection on truth rather than speculation offers patients the best opportunity for a curative response. The effective patient examination slowly and imperceptibly opens a window on, explores and confirms the conflicts of conscience. It discovers the whole truth about all aspects of the unique state of suffering. The inquiry views the symptoms within the context of the individual and the individual within the context of his environment and the universe, almost as if the illness was a Russian doll.

To locate the central disturbance, a state of stillness is required. The examination should calm troubled waters rather than stir them up. It is essential to observe shifts in patient body language that indicate a tender spot has been touched. Homœopathic practice is about gentle healing. Every question has the power to detonate past or present suffering and provoke a significant response. Tread carefully, as if crossing a minefield, lest the patient is unnecessarily disturbed. The goal is to identify and remove each mine, replace the earth around it, and then retreat in such a way no one knows you were there.

For example, if a patient reports experiencing some past atrocity or loss, don't drag them through that painful experience again by asking them to describe everything about it. An atrocity is an atrocity. A loss is a loss. Details of the atrocity itself are unnecessary. In homœopathy, it is the patient's responses and recurring patterns of reactions to events that are important because they individualise the character of the person and the degree and nature of the disturbance, and point directly to a particular remedy for the whole suffering.

To become a voyeur fascinated by each history is a temptation that is inappropriate and distracting. The correct patient examination is not psychotherapy. Rather than reopen an old wound and probe deeply and painfully, in homœopathy the object of the exercise is to skilfully encourage a wound to heal without reopening it.

If patients are to relax and not feel as though they are being hauled over red-hot coals or intently scrutinised, gentleness and consideration of their feelings are paramount. The proficient examination allows patients to stand at the edge of the ocean of distress, not to drown in its depths. Tenderly, and only for the briefest of moments, the practitioner glimpses and records the suffering and moves on.

It is essential to remember that as far as some patients are concerned, the reason they seek homœopathic help is for some physical symptom, e.g. a wart, eye, ear or digestive complaints.

It is certainly crucial to obtain information concerning intellectual and emotional changes experienced by patients, before during and after each symptom and how those changes relate to the whole illness. But it needs to be done without making patients feel that their suffering is being considered as 'all in the mind' insignificant, or that the interview is a form of disguised psychoanalysis.

To avoid patients experiencing this particular misunderstanding, unless the patient starts the story in the mental and emotional sphere, and doesn't know where to start, begin the patient examination line of inquiry somewhere other than the mind, such as the changes experienced in their General Physical Disposition. (See my plan of inquiry below).

Increased observation and sensory skills are demanded when patients are newborns, babies, children, adolescents, animals or the unconscious—individuals who, for one reason or another, are unable or unwilling to tell their story of suffering. That patient examination type may need to expand to include gathering relevant information from those around the patient. Unfortunately, relying on others for patient information often results in only a portion of the illness totality being discovered. Consequently, for these patients, the most suitable medicine is much harder to discover. In this case, instead of one, a series of different remedies might be required to achieve rapid restoration of health.

When the patient comes to the end of their story, the practitioner goes back through the report looking for information gaps and completes each symptom condition mentioned. This ensures that each tiny piece of information related to causation, sensation, location, side, extension, time and other modifying factors is gathered and recorded. This history record must faithfully represent every change from the patient's healthy state—spiritual, mind and body. It is those changes that form the basis of each prescription. A case may appear to be taken well, but there is uncertainty until the practitioner reviews the record and is able to identify the true image of the illness by its characteristic features.

The homœopathic patient examination is similar to going on a new hike. To avoid getting lost it is useful to carry and know how to use a map and compass and not rely on a GPS, which doesn't always work. Before starting out, it is necessary to understand how a compass works and review the map to get some idea of the landmarks to look for en route to your destination. It is wise to know where you are going and the safest, most direct route to take. Patient exhaustion might be an obstacle, so it best to avoid taking the scenic route.

To remind yourself what you need to know and to help you stay focused and on track, use Hahnemann's original case-taking instructions set down in *The Organon of Medicine* §83–§99 and create your own prompt sheet, including relevant 'open' questions to avoid yes or no answers. Mine lives on the left-hand side of my history-taking folio. To give you some idea of what is required here is an abbreviated version of my own history-taking interview structure including directions to the patient, open questions and information that must be covered, to provide a complete portrait of the disease.

Nicola's homœopathic patient exam prompt sheet

To make patients feel comfortable about what is going to happen I always start with this short introductory explanation:

Together we're going to paint a portrait of your illness. Without judgement of any kind regarding anything you say, I'm going to listen and record the information in your own words.

There are two common obstacles that must be removed: forgetfulness and medical terms.

Forgetfulness: Getting the whole illness history means working the memory unusually hard and it often fails. To help it along, let say we're in the middle of talking about bunions. Suddenly a memory of terrible constipation plops into your mind. Don't put it aside come right out with it there and then. If you put it away for later, it might be lost and it could be the most important piece of the puzzle. I'm taking verbatim notes so I can always bring us back to where we were before we made the detour.

Medical terms: To do a good job of providing information and trying to understand what's happening, some people may research the Internet and arrive at a self-diagnosis. Schooled in ordinary medicine, they use ordinary medical terms to explain and describe their illness. I need to understand your particular version of named conditions, so always use your own words and simple language to describe symptoms.

It's natural you might have questions as we go along. Ask them as they arise, and I will note them down, but I will postpone the answers until the end of the consult.

Patient examination starts

Please speak slowly so I may record your statements accurately.

If the patient can't seem to get started, pause for a short time to let them think, then say: Tell me about all the changes, discomfort you experienced when you became ill for the very first time, before you received any medical treatment.

Encourage the flow with: anything else?

After the patient stops their report, pause, then ask: what happened after that, bring me up to date.

Another way to get patients rolling is to say:

No matter how simple, complex, or even ridiculous it seems, describe in your own words how you are affected generally overall, for better or worse by:

- Air, inside/open air
- Heat or cold
- Desire for or aversion to motion, rest; exercise, walking, running, slowly/rapidly
- Weather, temperature changes
- Weakness, strength
- Pallor, flushing
- Time: hour, days, night, week, month, season
- Moon phases
- Light, darkness
- Travel
- Eating
- Before, during and after meals
- Time eat most, least
- Food cravings, aversions
- Drink cravings, aversions
- Thirst
- Taste
- Laying down, sitting, standing, bending
- Troublesome foods, drinks
- Puberty
- Adolescence
- Dizziness, fainting, loss of consciousness
- Fevers: heat chills, intensity, shivering, time of day/ circumstances, accompanying symptoms: perspiration including if any, colour, consistency, odour.
- Skin

- Pain: location, where it starts, where and how it goes, how it feels.

Then move to **Sleep-related disturbances and symptoms**. These are important because they are so closely related to the mind—the transfer from sleep to waking, from cerebrum to cerebellum.[80]

- Typical sleep pattern, beginning of sleep, during or after sleep, uncomfortable changes

- Preferred position, if known

- Gestures, sounds, movements, if known

- Sleepwalking or –talking

- Enduring, recurrent disturbing dreams

- Waking at night

- Sleepiness during the day

Then tiptoe towards the centre, The General Mental Emotional Disposition. (See *Formulating open questions* section above)

After patient or guardian stops, review each symptom, condition and where there are gaps, begin gathering information on the causation, sensation, location, duration, frequency, onset, what, where, when, how, modifying features of each symptom/condition.

To ensure nothing has been left out, I'm now going to conduct a head-to-toe check of the areas we've not already discussed. Tell me about any discomfort, changes you have experienced at any time during your life in the following regions of the body. (Go through each one separately; allow the patient time to think carefully about their answer):

- Changes in general: mental and physical disposition; sides affected; sleep.

- Head: hair, vertigo, Eyes and discharges, orbital regions, vision, headaches.

- Ears and discharges, hearing.

- Nose and discharges, smell.

- Face, cheeks, chin.

---

[80]   Dr. J.T. Kent, *Lectures on Homœopathic Philosophy*

- Mouth, teeth, gums, tongue, taste.

- Head pains.

- Neck [internal]: throat tonsils, thyroid, parathyroid, glands larynx and trachea, voice.

- Neck: skeleton, muscles, etc.

- Chest: breast, heart, respiration lungs, cough, mucous, expectoration.

- Digestion: oesophagus, stomach, abdomen, liver, rectum, anus.

- Elimination system: bowel movements (stools), urination, bladder, kidney, urethra, ureter and perspiration/skin.

- Females: Menstrual flow, present, ceased completely, age at onset, nature, run me through a typical cycle; pregnancy, childbearing, breast-feeding

- Males: genitals, semen and prostate gland.

- Describe any discomforts related to the sphere of sexual activity, function,sexually transmitted illnesses.

- Back, dorsal, lumbar, spine.

- Extremities shoulders, arms, hands, wrists, fingers, hips, legs, knees, ankles feet, toes

- Fevers, chills circulation, coldness/tingling/numbness.

Whether patients are humans or animals, with slight variations and obvious necessary omissions, the ideal rhythm of the effective interview is Inquire, Observe, Listen, Record and Recap, and goes something like this:

- Welcome and seat the patient.

- Gently set the patient at ease.

- Make yourself comfortable.

- Briefly explain the interview structure and goals.

- Observe each illness without prejudice.

- Remember to view each state of suffering as if it has never existed before in the world.

- Hold in your mind the progress of the patient's disorder from its beginning to its conclusion.

- Concentrate on collecting information about the *original natural illness* BEFORE medical treatment was administered.

- Ease up the window on the soul; release the suffering.

- Listen, observe and keep on track, record what you observe.

- Encourage more information: 'Is there anything else? Tell me more'.

- Wait a moment to ensure the patient has nothing more to say.

- Recap and clarify each trouble mentioned: possible cause, sensation, location, extension, modifying factors, etc.

- Expand the symptom image totality.

- Listen, observe and keep on track, record what you observe.

- Encourage.

- Listen, observe and keep on track, record what you observe.

- Recap and clarify as directed above.

Wrap up section

To encourage the release of the last drop of suffering, the last drop of information say something like: We are almost at the end of the interview. To help you, I need all the information I can get. Now is the time to think about whether there is anything else that might be important but requires a little more courage to report.

- Pause, wait for the response.

- Listen, observe, record, recap and clarify.

- Obtain family medical history.

Begin the final phase of the interview. To gain guidance on the central suffering say: I have learned a great deal about your illness. Please let me know which of those troubles bothers you the most.

Pause. Listen to the report, record and observe.

Remember, it is so easy to search for the medicine based on incorrect information. To avoid misunderstanding something extremely important, such as the central disturbance or the original causation of the illness, consider sharing your preliminary thoughts with the patient, say: I want to make sure I am correct in my understanding of your illness based on our discussion so far. Some people find this useful others do not want to know. Let me know if you are interested in learning what I have understood.

End of prompt sheet

Beware! In the homœopathic patient examination, it's never over until it's over.

Until you've waved the patient or guardian a fond farewell, the potential for the most precious information persists. Hand on the doorknob, out comes, 'Oh, I almost forgot. It's a small thing. I've always had it and don't suppose it has anything to do with anything … it's so trivial, but...' This is the moment the practitioner's memory is truly tested. Not wishing to interrupt the flow by walking back to pick up your exam record, you stand listening attentively until the patient finishes, and there it is: the most important clue to indicate the right remedy. Somehow you're going to have to formulate questions to get that last drop of information as you walk them out. You wave them off, dash back to your notes, still the mind and record that precious information, verbatim.

Ideally, regardless of species, all patients should leave the consulting room calmer than when they arrived—perhaps already in better health. A successful homœopathic patient examination lifts the spirits, leaves dignity firmly intact and the individual ready to face the world. The patient's facial expression and demeanour are telltale signs of how well things went. Where a patient appears exhausted, later the same day, give them a phone call to check how they're doing and if necessary smooth ruffled feathers. During the examination, it may happen that a practitioner combines attentive listening, empathy and health education so skilfully that a previously weakened vital force is markedly strengthened and the whole imbalance is corrected immediately. This could result in the fact that no homœopathic remedy is required at all. That's the ultimate in minimal medicine.

In my own practice, the aim is always to make a perfect first prescription. To give the patient my best effort, I need enough time to properly digest, organise and analyse the information received from the chronically ill patient, so I do not prescribe at the end of an examination. Several days later, after a great deal of careful deliberation I send the prescription, with the instruction to the patient to check in with me when they receive it and before taking it. I want to confirm there has been no improvement without medicine.

Where there is a dramatic improvement on all levels since the interview without any medicine, consider the patient examination released and roused the vital force sufficiently to finish the job it started. When that happens I enjoy a celebratory glass of Cremant du Bourgogne. Before administering what might be an unnecessary dose, I leave the patient alone without medicine waiting watchfully for the original symptoms to return and the right moment arises for the first prescription.

The next chapter discusses the quest for patient, illness and medicine similitude.

4

Medicine Selection Process

The homœopathic practitioner's primary duty must always be: *to select the first prescription properly and perfectly.* This chapter explains how to find the symptom-similar medicine most likely to cure. The tools required are a fully functioning brain with critical thinking ability, a dependable 'Repertory', which is an index of symptoms and their corresponding medicines, a reliable Materia Medica homœopathic medicine experiment knowledge base,[81] a pen and some paper.

Proper, proficient repertory use is indispensable to effective homœopathic practice. The case analysis, repertorial medicine selection methodology applied here is the rational, artistic, hierarchical methodology[82] which uses left and right sides of the human brain simultaneously, rather than a computer algorithm. Faithful to Hahnemann's remedy selection instructions articulated in The Organon of Medicine (§153), it offers clarity and provides consistency. Exquisite in its simplicity, this methodology takes a group of carefully selected symptoms that most precisely characterise and individualise the person and their suffering, and in just six thoughtful steps, the large group of

---

[81] Suggested texts: Dr. James Tyler Kent's *The Repertory of the Homœopathic Materia Medica* Hahnemann's two volume *Materia Medica Pura,* and two volume *The Chronic Diseases: Their Peculiar Nature and Their Homœopathic Cure*

[82] See Dr. J. T. Kent, *The Repertory of the Homœopathic Materia Medica,* three articles: Use of the Repertory; How to study the Repertory, and How to Use the Repertory.

remedies associated with each characteristic symptom is reduced and, a single remedy, or, as in the case of novice prescribers, a very small group of three or four medicines emerges.

Before the search for a medicine begins, the information gleaned from the patient examination must be carefully prepared for analysis. It is reckless to assume reams of notes indicate an effective patient examination. The patient has too much to lose if the prescription is incorrect.

The information gathered must be reviewed for its usefulness and relevance. It is important to look for and identify knowledge gaps, then go back to the patient and ask more questions to fill them in. The patient has too much to lose if the prescription is incorrect.

Efficient repertory work tends to identify all the remedies necessary in the entire course of treatment. The intellect must be focused to create a well-thought out plan of action. In that way the natural tendency for the mind to wander is interrupted. The practitioner is required to make sense of and use the mass of the illness history information gathered, and think clearly and deeply about each of a series of activities to be undertaken. Before opening the repertory proficient practitioners ask themselves two questions:

Exactly what is to be cured in each disease?

Exactly what is it I am looking for in the repertory?

To answer those questions, we need to isolate information that relates to the illness from its earliest beginning through to the moment the patient asked for help. The information retrieved relates to the chronology of symptoms and events from birth to present, which is organised into a timeline. Compilation of the Birth to Present Timeline does two important jobs. First, it indicates why, when and how each healthy person becomes ill and which inherent predisposition to illness is uppermost at a particular point in the patient's lifetime—progress of the disease. Then, it plots the curative route that the vital force is most likely to take as it retraces its steps back to the moment it was symptom-free, before it was disturbed, resolving previously unresolved conditions along the way.

This timeline is extremely important for another reason: Hahnemann instructs us to form a faithful picture of the disease, to grasp the permanent uncontaminated symptoms of the original natural illness and always to prescribe on the totality of individualising characteristic symptoms *before* the patient was treated with medicines or *after they have been discontinued for several days.*[83] When compiled accurately, the timeline is an essential treatment tool. It is referred to frequently, not only in progress reports but also when the time comes to consider changing medicines.

Next, the intelligent practitioner evaluates, rationalises and justifies the inclusion of each symptom to be used in the symptom picture totality and searched for in the repertory. According to Hahnemann, we're only looking for the *more striking, singular, uncommon, peculiar* (characteristic) signs and symptoms of the patient and the illness, because it is to these particular symptoms that the symptoms of the medicine must correspond.[84] Like whorls in a fingerprint, they are unique to each person—laden with details, including causation, sensation, location, side, extension, time and other modifying factors. They are both subjective symptoms: physical sensations and personal feelings; and objective symptoms: those observed by the practitioner. Characteristic individualising symptoms are things that make us hesitate and meditate.

A *Striking, Singular, Uncommon, Peculiar* (characteristic) symptom, is one that cannot be explained. It is one that is not common to disease but one that characterises the patient. They are so peculiar, so guiding and, therefore, so valuable that they must be ranked highest in order of importance. They are those symptoms, conditions and sensations the patient describes as 'odd' or 'weird'. For instance, in a chronic state of illness the patient is always very thirsty, but in an acute illness involving a burning fever, they are not thirsty.

Other examples of *striking, singular, uncommon and peculiar* (characteristic) symptoms are: 'My period (menstrual flow) only happens for one night each month.' Or 'I get these terrible bursting

---

[83] Dr. S. Hahnemann, *The Organon of Medicine*, Sixth edition, §91

[84] Ibid §153

pains in my head that go from one side to the other and the only thing that makes them better is when I punch my head with my fist.' Or 'Extreme thirst with an aversion to drinking water or any fluid.'

The easiest way to expose the *striking, singular, uncommon and peculiar* characteristics of the illness, the most useful information, is to identify and exclude useless information. Useless information can include: symptoms produced by iatrogenic disease, medicinal side effects, symptoms relating to pathology or the results of illness and symptoms that are specifically indicative of a particular disease or condition, e.g. breathing difficulties during asthma, skin eruptions in herpes. In the context of individualising a case for the purpose of medicine selection, which is common to any given disease is never *peculiar* or useful.

Common symptoms are excluded because they are observed in almost every disease and every medicine. They are more general and undefined, for example: loss of appetite, headache, debility, restless sleep, discomfort, heat with fever, sweat, vomiting, body ache and malaise. Common indications of fever are intense heat throughout the body, perspiration, a dry tongue and thirst. Suppose the patient describes swollen inflamed salivary glands and during the examination tells you not to press on them, as they are very sore. It is common for inflamed glands to be swollen sore, hard and tender when touched. Therefore, that information will not indicate a homœopathic remedy, unless there is some very striking feature or modifying factor related to it. Such as 'fever only at night', or 'fever without perspiration', or 'fever alternating with chills only after midnight without perspiration'.

Discarding the rubbish leaves the riches: the Totality of Individualising Characteristic Symptoms portrait of the illness.

To provide a working basis for each prescription and find the medicine or group of medicines that run through the totality of the characteristic symptoms, the individualising symptoms are then prioritised first to last from the most peculiar to the least peculiar to form a hierarchy of the most important symptoms. To do that, each characteristic symptom is examined individually and then valued for its perceived peculiarity. This process is often referred to as 'The Working'. Symptoms that affect the patient in general are valued and ranked higher than those that the affect the patient's parts. For example, symptoms related to the mental and emotional state take precedence over a pain in the thumb. This is where the characteristic symptom categories mentioned in the preceding chapter are used again.

Striking, Singular Uncommon and Peculiar (characteristic) symptoms: These are most highly valued because they are very odd. The great thing about these symptoms is that they stand out very clearly. They do not have to be contrived by the practitioner. If more than one very striking, peculiar symptom is identified, each symptom is valued and ranked separately according to its perceived peculiarity.

If no *striking, singular, uncommon and peculiar* (characteristic) symptoms are identified, search for and isolate 'those relating to changes in the state of the mind and disposition'.[85]

General Mental Emotional Disposition symptoms and modifying features, are valued, ranked and prioritised first to last in order of importance.

First: consider those characteristics and the causes relating to the innermost of the individual, any uncomfortable changes from the normal the state of mind. *Changes in longings, loves, desires, hates, aversions, antipathies, fears, dreads.*

Second: consider those characteristic symptoms that belong to *the rational, intellectual or reasoning faculties.* For example, where the patient cannot describe or narrate his symptoms or there is some mental confusion: loss of time sense, delirium or delusions, hallucinations that are not medicinally induced, which indicate changes in the ability to understand, changes in the intellectual portion of the individual. [86]

Third: consider *memory malfunction* symptoms. For example, difficulty concentrating, or making mistakes in writing and speaking. Of all the mind symptoms they are the most common symptoms.[87] They are less important, unless the central disturbance happens to be 'extreme forgetfulness', then its level

---

[85] Dr. S. Hahnemann, *The Organon of Medicine,* Sixth edition §213

[86] Dr. J. T. Kent, *Repertory of the Homœopathic Materia Medica.*

[87] Ibid

of importance increases proportionally and it becomes a characteristic symptom.

Fourth in line for consideration are *sleep disturbance symptoms and their modifying features*. These are important because they are so closely related to the mind.[88] And sleep is the bridge between the active and resting mind.

With the General Mental Disposition characteristic morbid changes isolated we turn our attention to the:

General Physical Disposition symptoms and modifying features. These are the physical symptoms related to the blood, colour of discharge, and bodily aggravation and amelioration, that include the whole being, as well as desire for open air, desire for heat, cold air, for rest, for motion, which may be only a desire or may bring a general feeling of amelioration—symptoms and modifying features that are related to how the entire being is affected. It should be understood a circumstance that makes the whole being feel better or worse is of much greater importance than when the same circumstances only affect the painful part. However, these are often quite opposite, e.g. the patient as a whole has a lack of vital heat, yet the suffering part is worsened by heat. An important place must be given to the time of day, night or season every symptom occurs. Priority is always allocated to *blood, colour of discharges* from ulcers, uterus during menstruation, from ears and from other parts, as those are very closely related to the operation of the vital force. [89]   Information concerning flow, consistency and factors that worsen or ameliorate discharges is important. For example: pus indicates septic states the vital force is severely weakened; clear fluid indicates the vital force is less severely weakened. Information concerning odour, colour, consistency, hot/ cold, flow, location[s], the effect of the discharge on on body e.g. rawness, discolouration and factors that worsen or ameliorate discharges is important. It is common for blood to clot; it is peculiar for blood not to clot.

---

[88] Ibid

[89] Ibid

More examples of General Physical Disposition symptoms related to the whole individual are:

- The things described by the patient as 'I do so and so. Dr., I feel so and so, I have so much thirst, I am so chilly in every change of weather, I suffocate in a warm room,' etc.[90]

- Sensitivity to open air, heat, light, food, fluids, night, day, season

- Desire for, or aversion to, rest or motion or any of the above mentioned

- Weakness or skin pallor

- For females: how affected before, during and after menstrual flow

- Eating: how affected before, during and after

- Rectal/urinary evacuation: how they are affected before, during and after

Up to this point, the *striking, uncommon* characteristic symptoms and everything and anything that belongs to the whole person in general, everything that indicates he feels so and so, she suffers so and so, the *general mental, emotional and general physical disposition* characteristics have been singled out for study and valued.

In the next step, the case analysis moves from identifying the *general* to identification of the *particular* more striking, singular, uncommon and peculiar (characteristic) signs and symptoms—those related to a part, region or organ of the body, and of the extremities; the patient describes 'my' head, kidney, breast, leg, arm, breathing, etc.[91] a region, affinity, location, symptoms that extend in one direction or another, one part of the body to another and their modifying features.

In six steps, the vast mass of information recorded while taking the history has been correctly valued and significantly reduced. A striking recognisable likeness of the illness has emerged with all the features faithfully represented, and each given its correct prominence within the context of the whole portrait. The symptom totality portrait of the

---

[90] Ibid

[91] Dr. J. T. Kent, *Repertory of the Homœopathic Materia Medica.*

illness has been carefully organised to represent the patient from innermost to outermost, Generals to Particulars. Any remedy correctly worked out this way should agree with and fit the patient, their symptoms, parts and modalities.[92] A medicine with the power to induce the greatest number of symptoms similar to those experienced is likely to be found.

Ideally, there should be a characteristic symptom in each of the above categories. However, due to a) the uniqueness of patient and illness, and b) the need to avoid all speculation about a symptom or condition, parts of the symptom totality portrait might be missing, which reduces the potential for selecting a suitable remedy. To stand a chance of finding the correct medicine, the smallest Totality of Characteristic Individualising Symptoms picture of the illness must include at least one General Mental, Emotional Disposition characteristic symptom, one General Physical Disposition characteristic symptom and one or more striking Particular Characteristic Symptom.

Using the examples of strange rare and peculiar symptoms mentioned above as well as those of 'pneumonia' patient, the information is prioritised and arranged to form a hierarchy of symptoms like this:

Striking, Singular Uncommon and Peculiar symptoms: Menstrual flow for one night only every month. Head pains, bursting, ameliorated by banging head against something hard.

General Mental Emotional Disposition symptoms: 'the other thing is I just want to be by myself. That's strange because normally I love people around me. I can't get enough of them. I just can't lie or sit still. If I do, I get very anxious.'

Sleep Related Symptoms: None identified.

General Physical Disposition Symptoms: 'Everything is much worse after midnight—the pain, the coughing, everything. I have so much pain in my body, so I move about, even though when I begin to move, the pain is so much worse; but if I keep moving around, it gets better. That's why I go from the bed to the chair and back again and move around in the bed. By the

---

[92] Dr. J. T. Kent, *Repertory of the Homœopathic Materia Medica*

way, the pains move around from one part of me to another. I never know where they are going to be next. I don't want to drink water or any fluid.'

Particular Symptoms: a bright red triangular area at the tip of the tongue, the eyes are only partly open, the arms are drawn up to the chest, and the face is deathly pale with beads of perspiration on the chin. An odour of rotting flesh exudes from the mouth.

Common Symptoms: 'It came on after I got chilled in a downpour.'

To find the medicine, the practitioner takes each characteristic symptom and begins to search for it in the Repertory where symptoms are organised under regions of the body—mind, head, back—and arranged alphabetically according to subsections: sides, time, modifications, extensions. If the patient's exact words cannot be found, the practitioner looks for synonyms or phrases that most closely represent the patient's descriptions. For example, where the patient complains of a 'dead' leg, medicines producing that symptom will be found under the word 'numbness' medicines that produce the feeling that the head is 'big' will be found under the rubric 'head, sensation as if enlarged'.

Using the individualisation hierarchy as the guide, each symptom is taken in order, and searched for in the repertory. In this instance:

Symptom 1: Menstrual flow one night only every month.

Symptom 2: Head pain bursting, banging head against something hard ameliorates.

The group of medicines related to symptom 1 is compared with the group of remedies related to symptom 2. The only remedies written down are those that are *common to both groups of remedies.* The rest are eliminated. This action is repeated with each symptom. When a rubric cannot be found for a symptom, it is necessary to halt the search for that symptom and begin to search for a rubric for the next symptom on the list. Through this process of elimination, a group of remedies runs through the totality of symptoms until a single remedy, or three, or four emerges. The final arbiter is always the medicine experiment knowledge base. The practitioner carefully reviews the information related to each medicine to verify which one shares the greatest number of symptoms similar to both the medicinal symptoms and the totality of characteristic symptoms experienced.

Let's apply the method to a couple of Hahnemann's simple cases.[93] The repertory used is Dr. J. T. Kent's *Repertory of the Homœopathic Materia Medica*. You will observe, from a mass of symptoms and medicines, the single most suitable remedy quickly emerges.

Hahnemann's first sample case

A washer woman, somewhere about forty years old, had been unable to earn her bread for more than four weeks when she consulted me on the first day of September 1815.

The symptoms:

- On any movement, especially every step, and worst (sic) on making a false step, she has a shoot in the pit of the stomach that comes as she avers, every time from the left side.
- When she lies down she feels quite well, then she has not pain anywhere neither in the side nor in the pit of the stomach.
- She cannot sleep after three o'clock in the morning.
- She relishes her food, but when she has eaten a little she feels sick.
- Then the water collects in her mouth and runs out of it, like the water brash.
- She has frequent empty eructation (airless, belching, burping) after every meal.
- Her temper is passionate, disposed to anger.
- When the pain is severe, she is covered with perspiration.
- Her menstrual flow is regular and occurred two weeks ago.

In other respects, her health is good.

In discussing this case Hahnemann says: For the convenience of treatment, we require merely to jot down after each symptom all medicines which can produce such a symptom with tolerable accuracy,

---

[93] Dr. S. Hahnemann, *Materia Medica Pura,*

expressing them by a few letters: e.g., Ferr. Chin. Rheum. Puls, and to also consider the circumstances under which they occur, which have a determining influence on our choice. Continue in the same way with all the other symptoms, noting by what medicine each is excited; from the list so prepared, we shall be able to perceive which, among the medicines, homœopathically covers the most of the symptoms present, especially the most peculiar and characteristic ones—and this is the remedy sought for.

Hahnemann identifies the following symptoms as characteristic indications of a particular remedy and ranks them in order of their peculiarity:

Striking, singular, uncommon and peculiar characteristic symptoms:

Shooting (pain) in the pit of the stomach on making a false step.

General mental, emotional disposition:

Her temper is passionate, disposed to anger.

General physical disposition modifying feature:

No pain anywhere, neither in the side nor in the pit of the stomach during rest and when lying down.

Particulars:

When she has eaten a little she feels sick.

After eating, empty eructation (belch of wind only).

To find the medicine most likely to cure, the first symptom to search for in the repertory is the:

Striking, singular, uncommon and peculiar symptom:

Shooting in the pit of the stomach, on making a false step.

There will be a group of medicines next to that symptom.

I write out that grouping in its entirety, using the abbreviated form of the remedy names: Bry., Puls.

I search in the repertory for the next symptom:

General Mental, Emotional Disposition:

Disposed to anger

There will be a group of remedies next to this symptom. To find the medicine most likely to cure, I must write out only the remedies that are common to both groupings, and eliminate all remedies that are not in both groupings:

I am left with: Bry. Puls.

I search the repertory for the next symptom:

General Physical Disposition, the modifying feature:

There is no pain anywhere, when resting or lying down.

There will be a group of remedies next to this symptom. I write out only the remedies that are common to both groupings. Remedies that are not in both groupings are eliminated:

The remedy that remains is: Bryonia

Usually a group of five or ten remedies remains at this point, but already at this point in this sample case, only *one* remedy remains: Bryonia.

To confirm accuracy of the selection, the analysis must be continued and completed.

I continue searching the repertory for the next symptom:

General Physical Disposition, the modifying feature:

When she has eaten a little, she feels sick.

There will be a group of remedies next to this symptom.

I eliminate remedies that are not in both groupings, and write out only the remedies that are in both groupings:

I'm left with: Bryonia.

I search the repertory for the remaining symptoms.

Particulars:

After eating, empty (without gas, wind) eructation (belching).

There will be a group of remedies next to this symptom.

I eliminate medicines that are not in both groupings and write out only those that are common to both groupings:

The remedy that remains is: Bryonia.

It is the only remedy that ran through all the symptoms.

Having conducted so many experiments with medicines and documented their effects, Hahnemann's knowledge of medicinal symptoms was profound. In the case described above, he considers the medicinal symptom image of Bryonia and its symptom-similarity with the illness experienced and prescribes a single dose of Bryonia.

He asks the patient to return in 48 hours. She never returns.

Hahnemann told a friend of his who was half-converted to homœopathy that he knew she would be completely cured. The friend expressed his doubts. To allay the doubt, (and breaking the rule of patient confidentiality!) Hahnemann gave his friend the patient's name and address and told him to go and see for himself. He did. In response to the question why didn't you go back? The patient answered:

> What was the use of my going back? The very next day I was quite well, I returned to my washing. The day after that I was well, I am still well. I am extremely obliged to the doctor, but people like us have no time to leave off our work; and for three weeks previously my illness had prevented me from earning a living.

Hahnemann's second sample case

W, a weakly, pale man of forty-two years who was constantly kept at his desk by his business, complained to me on 27 December 1815, that he had been ill for five days.

The symptoms:

- The first evening, without cause, he became sick and giddy with much eructation.
- The following night (about 2 a.m.) sour vomiting.
- The subsequent nights violent eructations experienced.
- Today also sick; eructation of fetid and sourish taste experienced.
- He felt as if food lay crude and undigested in his stomach.
- In his head he felt vacant, hollow and gloomy and as if sensitive therein.
- The least noise was disagreeable to him.
- He is of a mild, soft, patient disposition.

In discussing this case, Hahnemann does not perceive the existence of striking, strange, rare, peculiar symptoms. Therefore, this case analysis repertory search starts with the:

General Mental Emotional Disposition symptoms:

Mildness

Sensitive to noise

Writing out only the remedies common to both groupings they are (in abbreviated form):

Acon. Ambr. Arn. Ars. Ars-i. Asar. Aur. Bell. Bor. Cact. Calc. Caps. Carb-an. Caust. Chel. Cic. Cocc. Hell. Ign. Iod. Kali-c. Kali-p. Lyc. Mang. Mosch. Nat-a. Nat-c. Nat-m. Nit-ac. Op. Ph-ac. Phos. Puls. Rhus-t. Sep. Sil. Stann. Zinc.

General Physical Disposition:

Vertigo with eructation

Writing out only the remedies common to both groupings, remedies that remain: Nat-m, Puls

Particulars:

Discharges from orifices always take priority because they indicate the innermost operation of the vital force of nature,[94] so:

Stomach, vomiting sour

Remedies that remain: Nat-m. Puls

The next particular characteristic symptom should be:

Stomach indigestion

Remedies that remain: Nat-m. Puls

The next symptom should be:

Stomach eructation night

Remedies that remain: Pulsatilla

Discussing the case, Hahnemann writes:

> This patient could not be cured by anything in a more easy, certain, and permanent manner than by Pulsatilla, which was homœopathic to this case. Accordingly, it was given to him immediately … in the evening. The next day he was free of all ailments, his digestion was restored, and a week thereafter, as he told me, he remained free from complaint and quite well.

At the end of a repertory analysis, when more than one medicine remains in contention, the one that is most likely to ignite the vital force's curative response is the one with the greatest number of characteristic individualising symptoms similar to those experienced by the patient.

---

[94] Dr. J.T Kent, *Repertory of the Homœopathic Materia*, Article: Use of the Repertory

Therefore, before choosing and administering any medicine, its patient—illness similitude must always be properly confirmed. The practitioner studies two things very carefully: the exact words and phrases used by the patient to describe their suffering, and the detailed descriptions of suffering documented in the homœopathic *Materia Medica*. The information must be studied until there is certainty about the similarity between both descriptions, and absolutely *no doubt* exists about which medicine shares the greatest number of symptoms similar to those experienced by the patient. The correct medicine must run through *all* the characteristic symptoms of the case. The clearer, more peculiar and more characteristic individualising symptoms there are in the case and the greater the number of similar characteristic symptoms shared between illness and medicine there are, the greater the likelihood that the medicine will suit the patient and illness.

Unskilled in valuing the characteristic nature of each symptom, The Working of some practitioners may include lots of common, less characteristic symptoms of the patient and illness. A large group of remedies runs through all the symptoms. The larger the group of remedies remaining at the end of The Working, the more likely it is that the practitioner has either misunderstood what is to be cured in the illness, or not taken sufficient time to think carefully about and discriminate between which symptoms should be included in the analysis and which should be excluded. That lack of discrimination translates to an inability to differentiate between medicines and much more time trying to decide which remedy to select. To avoid doing that, they are more likely to depend solely on artificial intelligence—they start at the top of a computer-generated list of medicines and, disregarding the potential for every medicine to alter the person's state of health, work their way down the list administering one medicine after another, until by chance they hit upon one that induces improved health.

Patient recovery hinges on practitioner accuracy in selecting the first and each subsequent remedy and dose. Patients are dependent on practitioner conscientiousness and knowledge related to what is to be cured in each case, whether the practitioner searches both homœopathic *Materia Medica* and *repertory*, practitioner repertory searching skills, and the reliability of information contained in both books. Over time, many different versions of these texts have been created, along with different criteria for excluding and including certain medicines. As the accuracy of that information varies, so must the accuracy of medicine selection.

> This laborious, sometimes very laborious, search for and selection of the homœopathic remedy most suitable in every respect to each morbid state, is an operation which, notwithstanding all the admirable books for facilitating it, still demands the study of the original sources themselves and at the same time a great amount of circumspection and serious deliberation, which have their best reward in the consciousness of having faithfully discharged our duty.[95]

For consistency and accuracy, of the two precision instruments used to find the right medicine, Hahnemann considers his four volumes of homœopathic *Materia Medica (Materia Medica Pura,* and *The Chronic Diseases: Their Peculiar Nature and Their Homœopathic Cure)* to be most reliable because they contain the original unmodified detailed healthy person and medicine experiment information. He says repertories:

> …Are only intended to give light hints as to one or another medicine that might be selected, but they can never dispense him from making the research from the first fountain heads. He who does not take the trouble of treading this path in all critical and complicated diseases, and, indeed, with all patience and intelligence, but contents himself with vague hints of the repertories in the choice remedy, and who thus quickly dispatches one patient after the other, does not deserve the honorable title of a genuine Homœopath, but is rather to be called a bungler, who on that account has continually to change his remedies until the patient loses patience; and as his ailments have of course only been aggravated he must leave this aggravator of diseases, whereby the art itself suffers discredit instead of the unworthy disciple of art.[96]

Having selected the correct medicine, the next challenge is selecting the proper dose and proper intervals for each patient.

---

[95] Dr. S. Hahnemann, *The Organon of Medicine,* Sixth edition, §148, F/n 108.

[96] Dr. S. Hahnemann, *The Chronic Diseases: Their Peculiar Nature and Their Homœopathic Cure*

5

Proper Dose Selection

For a homœopathic medicine to have the desired, gentle, efficacious effect, and to mitigate the risks of increasing suffering —no matter how short lasting—it is essential that the same degree of careful thought applied to choosing the most suitable homœopathic medicine is also applied to selection of the most suitable amount/potency and dosing regimen.

Cure using homœopathy always depends on shared similitude between symptoms produced by the illness and those produced by a medicine, plus shared similitude between the dose and the proportion of strength with which the vital force still prevails in the patient. It cannot be said that selection of the correct medicine is finished until the potency and dosage have been decided. The perfect homœopathic prescription penetrates to the centre of the disturbance, works in union with the vital force, boosting its remaining power, enabling it to free itself from harm and restore lasting balance throughout the body. The proper dose must be just sufficient—no more, no less—to engage the vital force in repairing the damage its struggles caused and transform illness into health, without overwhelming it. The more susceptible the patient is to the medicine and dose, the less resistance to the medicine will be encountered, and the gentler and faster the recovery. A useful rule to follow is, *the closer the resmblance between symptoms of the natural disease and symptoms produced by the medicine, the LESS medicine is required.*

To select the proper smallest dose of medicine, the following factors are carefully weighed:

- The proportion of strength or weakness of the vital force that still prevails in the patient.
- The patient's susceptibility, their ability to react
- The centre of the disturbance or seat of the disease
- Location and intensity of each symptom experienced
- The nature of the disease being treated (acute, chronic)
- The stage of the disease (beginning, middle, end)
- Previous treatment of the disease
- Whether the patient is receiving mainstream and homœopathic medicine concurrently.
- Presence of obstacles to cure, including repeated exposure to avoidable harmful influences

Depending on the strength or weakness of the vital force at a given moment, the central disturbance manifests in the spiritual, intellectual, emotional or physical spheres and the degree of the patient's strength or weakness. Where the intensity of suffering is experienced in the interior of the body—energy, mental, emotional, vital organs, body fluids, etc.—the vital force is understood to be extremely weak. At this point, it is insufficient to resist or to protect the inner regions of the body from harm and is unable to push the disturbance to the peripheral regions. Where most of the suffering is experienced in the less vital regions— muscles, skeleton, skin, etc.—the vital force is understood to be somewhat stronger, sufficient enough to keep the central disturbance in the outer regions but insufficient to completely expel the harm and restore health.

In homœopathic practice, individualisation between potencies provides an additional element of accuracy and success, enabling us to treat certain cases that we otherwise could not reach.

Hahnemann's two different dosage scales are LM/Q and 'c' centesimal. This is discussed in greater detail in the previous

Chapter 1, under the heading Smallest dose: dilution and potentiation.

In Hahnemann's view the LM/Q potency scale is the perfected minimal, most efficient, most powerful yet mildest homœopathic medicine dose. It simplifies proper dose selection enormously because it eliminates practitioner confusion associated with centesimal potency decisions regarding whether to select low, medium or high potencies. Exactly as Hahnemann intended, the LM/Q potency avoids the overreactions commonly produced by giving too high centesimal doses. The LM/Q dosing methodology must never be confused with the so-called 'drop dosing' prescriber divergence.

LM/Q dosing is suitable for the ailing vital force of all ages, conditions and stages of illness, and especially for:

- Gross pathology
- Mainstream medicine or homœopathic medically mismanaged individuals.
- Drug and alcohol abuse
- Continuing intentional excess or deprivation of life-sustaining elements such as food, air, water, heat or light
- Individuals suffering acute or deep-seated, longstanding, complicated disorders such as those affecting the brain, respiratory system or skin, and which have been previously treated with strong mainstream medications and surgical intervention.
- Borderline curable states where the revival of a severely weakened vital force is doubtful
- Individuals who are naturally highly sensitive
- Individuals suffering from medicine-induced hypersensitivity
- Individuals whose illness demands continued life-sustaining substances such as insulin in the treatment of diabetes concurrent with homœopathic treatment.
- Individuals who seek to reduce dependency on mainstream medication.

- Individuals suffering long-term fatigue, indicating a severely weakened vital force
- Deep-seated, longstanding or urgent-need mood swings.
- Conditions arising during times of psychological and physiological transition, e.g. puberty, adolescence, menopause, ageing.
- Individuals burdened by 'maintaining' causes of illness that for various reasons cannot be eliminated such as famine, overwork, domestic violence, imprisonment, etc.

To enable patients to learn how to use the LM/Q potency to best advantage, at the beginning of dosing, at least for the first month, practitioner time needs to be spent talking to patients to confirm or deny improvement is under way, and to ensure any dosing adjustments that may be required are made promptly.

At the beginning of using the LM/Q dosing, some patients may still experience false starts, setbacks and tough days. This often depends on the nature and degree of previous medical mismanagement, the extent to which the vital force has been weakened and the complexity of suffering experienced. Provided the practitioner selects the most suitable symptom-similar remedy and proper dosing intervals, and monitors patient responses at appropriate intervals, such stuttering progress is efficiently minimised. Administered properly, LM/Q doses gently fan the embers of the patient's vital force into an intermittent spark, until that spark multiplies and coalesces into a forceful, self-sustaining flame allowing recovery to pick up pace.

When LM/Q doses are administered to individuals who are ill but have *not* been medically mismanaged they tend to move more continuously and rapidly along the road to recovery with very little interruption and minimal or no overreaction.

The full LM/Q potency scale ranges from LM/Q#01 to LM/Q#30.

The dosing rules are as follows:

- *Always* start at potency LM/Q#01 and ascend the scale.[97]

---

[97] Dr. S. Hahnemann, *The Organon of Medicine*, Sixth edition, §246

- LM/Q potency pellets are *always* dissolved in water before administration.

Hahnemann wanted LM/Q dose administration tools to be simple. Therefore, he used tablespoons, teaspoons and coffee spoons as measuring devices. The effect on patients of *teaspoon or coffee spoon daily doses* versus tablespoon medicinal doses is different. It is very useful for reducing overreactions that might occur in children, naturally hypersensitive individuals or individuals who have been rendered artificially hypersensitive to all medicines by prolonged use of very powerful mainstream medications.

Hahnemann's LM/Q medicinal solution consists of a pellet or globule (and it is rarely necessary to use more than one globule) from the vial LM/Q#01 dissolved in 7, 8, 15, 20, 30 or 40 tablespoons of water with the addition of some alcohol or a piece of charcoal in order to preserve it. In the following instructions, the words 'succussion' and 'agitation' refer to downward strokes of the arm.

For medicinal solutions made in 15, 20, 30 or 40 tablespoons of water, the dosing instructions are:

> The medicinal solution is potentised again: (with perhaps 8, 10, 12 succussions) from which we give the patient one or (increasingly) several teaspoonful doses, in long lasting disease daily or every second day, in acute diseases every two to six hours and in very urgent cases every hour or oftener. Thus in chronic disease, every correctly chosen homœopathic medicine, even those whose action is of long duration, may be repeated daily for months with ever increasing success.[98]

> If the solution is used up (in seven to fifteen days) and the same medicine is still indicated, it is necessary to make up a new medicinal solution using one or (though rarely) several pellets of a higher potency [LM/Q #02] with which we continue so long as the patient experiences continued improvement without encountering one or another complaint he never had before in his life.[99]

---

[98] Dr. S. Hahnemann, *The Organon of Medicine*, Sixth edition, §248, including Footnote 134.

[99] Ibid

However, to avoid the need for a large quantity of water, Hahnemann recommends making the medicinal solution using a pellet or globule from the vial LM/Q#01 dissolved in 7–8 tablespoons of water, which is equivalent to 4 fl. oz. /110ml.

The dosing method for that medicinal solution is as follows:

> ... *After thorough succussion of the vial* [with perhaps 8, 10, 12 succussions] take from it one tablespoon and put it in a glass of water, (containing about 7 to 8 tablespoons of water) this is *stirred thoroughly* then give a [teaspoon] dose to the patient'.[100]

> As described above, in long lasting disease the patient may be given one or several teaspoonful doses daily or every second day; in acute diseases every two to six hours and in very urgent cases every hour or oftener.

> Where the patient is unusually excited and sensitive, a teaspoonful of this [first glass] solution may be put in a second glass of water, thoroughly stirred, and teaspoonful doses or more may be given. There are patients of so great sensitivity that a third or fourth glass similarly prepared may be necessary.

> When the first bottle is used up, then a second bottle containing the next ascending LM/Q potency pellet or globule is prepared and the dosing procedure for the first bottle is continued, and so on up the scale.[101] So long as the patient experiences continued improvement, and does not experience one or another complaint that he never had before in his life, i.e. new symptoms, the patient continues to dose daily or every second day.[102]

When advising patients on LM/Q potencies to dose daily, it is important to avoid making a common serious error. Homœopathic daily dosing of medicine should never be confused with the routine daily dosing according to ordinary medical practice. When using either centesimal or LM/Q homœopathic dosing methods, the rule is: *to ensure repeated doses do not injure the patient, the patient is*

---

[100] Ibid F/n 134.

[101] Dr. S. Hahnemann, *The Organon of Medicine*, Sixth edition,§248

[102] Ibid §248

monitored for changes after each dose of medicine and the patient is directed to
report any worsening effects of the medicine immediately.

In urgent care treatment, depending on the severity or life-threatening nature of the illness, intervals between doses and patient evaluation progress reports may be five, ten, twenty or thirty minutes and so on. At the beginning of treating chronic illness using the LM/Q method, in order to find the optimal dosing period for each patient, it is wise and essential to monitor patients for changes at three-, five- or seven-day intervals for the first four weeks. The LM/Q dosing instruction to patients should be:

> *Begin dosing as directed: for urgent care illness report in 5, 10, 20 minutes. For chronic*
> *illnesses report in (three, five or seven) days, but if you feel unwell in any way at all at*
> *any time for any reason during that period e.g. earlier that three, five or seven days, stop*
> *dosing immediately and report for evaluation, explanation and further instructions.*

In that way, patients avoid experiencing an unrecognised non-curative response for too long without a necessary dosing adjustment being made. Monitoring at proper intervals confirms patients experience continued improvement without the need to adjust the dose. Following this protocol also allows patients to become familiar with the dosing method and have confusions quickly clarified. See Chapter 10 for detailed analyses of vital force responses to LM/Q dosing.

The safest general rules for the centesimal potency selection, based upon firm adherence to the laws of homœopathy and practised by practitioners closest to Hahnemann are as follows:

- Give one remedy at a time.
- Give a single dose.
- Give the first dose in a moderate potency with a tendency to go higher at proper intervals.

Where the vital force is strong and, able to keep venting the disturbance in a variety of ways including onto the surface areas, patients experience lots of symptoms with great intensity. The clearer, more peculiar and more characteristic individualising symptoms there are in the case and the greater the number of similar symptoms shared between illness and medicine, the higher the degree of patient susceptibility to the medicine is. Where the symptoms of a case clearly indicate one remedy and the characteristic symptoms of that remedy correspond most closely to the characteristic symptoms of the patient and illness, that remedy is usually prescribed in the moderate 30c to higher range of potency, depending on the prescriber's degree of confidence in the accuracy of their prescription.

Susceptibility to the medication is considered to be low in the following circumstances: where the symptoms are not clearly developed and there is an absence or scarcity of characteristic individualising symptoms; where gross pathology exists; where the weakened vital force is unable to expel the disturbance outward onto the surface areas; where there are few physical symptoms; discomfort exists proportionately more at the innermost levels and less at the outermost levels; or where two or three remedies seem equally indicated.

It is wise to be very cautious about using the lower 3c, 6c to 12c potencies. They should be repeated very rarely. There are several reasons for this: lower centesimal potencies are less dilute, they contain more crude substance—a larger amount of it—and consequently they are closer to mainstream medicine physiological drug doses and therefore they are more likely to induce a lasting aggravation of the existing symptoms as well as producing their own pathogenetic symptoms. These medicinally produced symptoms might commingle with the existing symptoms of the illness being treated, and thereby increase rather than reduce suffering.

> Several times I have seen patients on repeated doses of the right remedy in low potency make no improvement, simply because their susceptibility to that *potency*—not to that remedy by any means—had

been exhausted. I have taken such patients and without changing the remedy but simply the potency got a curative result.[103]

Hahnemann says it is dangerous to prescribe *too strong a dose* of medicine, even if it is quite homœopathically chosen for the disease being treated. In spite of the inherent beneficial character of its nature, it must prove injurious by its mere magnitude, because of its homœopathic similarity of action, and by the too strong impression it makes on the vital force and upon those parts of the body which are most sensitive and already most affected by the natural disease.[104] He explains why:

> For this reason, a medicine, even though it may be homœopathically suited to the case of disease, does harm in every dose that is too large, and in strong doses it does more harm the greater its homœopathicity and the higher the potency selected, and it does much more injury than any equally large dose of a medicine that is unhomœopathic and in no respect adapted to the morbid state (allopathic).

> Too large doses of an accurately chosen homœopathic medicine, and especially when frequently repeated, bring about much trouble as a rule. They put the patient not seldom in danger of life or make his disease almost incurable. They do indeed extinguish the natural disease so far as the sensation of the life principle is concerned and the patient no longer suffers from the original disease from the moment the too strong dose of the homœopathic medicine acted upon him but he is in consequence more ill with the similar but more violent medicinal *disease which* is most difficult to destroy.[105]

The best time to take the medicine in treatment of **chronic** illness is as follows:

> The remedy is best received by the vital force early in the morning before breakfast, without drinking or eating anything within half an hour or a whole hour.

---

[103] Dr. J.T. Kent, *Lectures on Homœopathic Philosophy*, & Kent's *New Remedies, Clinical Cases, Lesser Writings, Aphorisms and Precepts,* compiled by Dr. W.W. Sherwood

[104] Dr. S. Hahnemann, *The Organon of Medicine*, Sixth edition, §275

[105] Dr. S. Hahnemann, *The Organon of Medicine*, Sixth edition, §276

It should be taken by itself, dry and allowed to dissolve on the tongue, or moistened with two or three drops of water on a spoon. Ideally, after the dose the patient should keep perfectly quiet for at least a full hour, but without going to sleep (sleep delays the beginning of the medicine action). During this hour, as indeed throughout treatment, the patient must avoid all disagreeable excitement. Immediately after taking the dose, the patient should not strain the mind either by reading, or computing, by writing or by conversations requiring thought.[106]

Given that most mornings we need to hit the ground running and keep going, the best most patients can do to comply with Hahnemann's instructions is to take the medicine on waking and wait twenty minutes before brushing teeth, drinking or eating breakfast. Even with these constraints, the medicine is effective.

Females should avoid taking the medicine shortly before the menstrual flow is expected, or during the flow; but if necessary [e.g. the patient is suffering profoundly] it may be given four days, i.e., about ninety-six hours, after the menstrual flow has started.

Breast feeding infants never receive medicine: instead, the mother receives the infant's remedy, and through the breast milk it acts on the child very quickly, mildly and beneficially.[107]

For **urgent acute** illness the time to dose is as follows:

Administer the remedy quickly after it has been selected, or if it is a violent spasm or a fever with a particular sequence of heat and chills, quickly after the paroxysm.

At that moment, a small pellet of one of the highest dynamisations of a medicine is laid dry on the tongue until it dissolves, or (extremely useful in treatment of unconscious or highly sensitive patients) moderate smelling of an opened vial containing pellets in the potency selected, proves to be the smallest and weakest dose with the shortest duration of effect. This dosage method is particularly appropriate in slight acute illness, where the patient is naturally excitable.

---

[106] Dr. S. Hahnemann, The *Chronic Diseases: Their Peculiar Nature and Their Homœopathic Cure.*

[107] Dr. S. Hahnemann, *The Chronic Diseases: Their Peculiar Nature and Their Homœopathic Cure.*

In acute and very urgent illness, according to the degree and nature of suffering experienced, it may be that the medicine is required to act more strongly, or rapid repetition of the medicine may be necessary.

In which case, it must be stirred until it has dissolved, in seven to twenty tablespoonfuls of water, and a tablespoon portion of the mixture taken at a time, every hour, or every half-hour; two, three, four or six hours. In taking the same medicine repeatedly, the power of the dose must be altered slightly, before each dose. To effect the alteration every time, before each dose, the container should be shaken vigorously five or six times.

Weak patients and children should be given one or two tea or coffee spoonfuls as a dose.[108]

In the treatment of chronic illness—where there is uncertainty about whether the vital force has completely finished responding to a very high dose of a medicine that has proved extremely beneficial, coupled with uncertainty about moving to the next higher potency that might be too much—one dose of same potency given in the extra dilution and agitation described by Hahnemann is especially useful. The vital force will receive it without resistance and use it for a little longer until it reaches the end of its curative power. When the existing symptoms of the case return, there is then more certainty about moving to the next higher dose.

Hahnemann considers the widespread recommendation to give patients several dry doses of the same remedy and potency to take with them, so that they may take a dose at certain intervals or as needed without considering whether any repetition may injure the patient, to be negligent empiricism unworthy of a homœopathic practitioner.[109]

He instructs that doses of homœopathic medicines should be repeated *only after the practitioner has carefully re-examined the patient* and is convinced that the first dose proved beneficial. After

---

[108] Ibid

[109] Dr. S. Hahnemann, *The Chronic Diseases: Their Peculiar Nature and Their Homœopathic Cure*

improvement stops, and when the patient relapses, the intensity of the returning symptoms indicates that a new dose of the same remedy is required to calm them. That first dose of medicine slightly increased the power of the vital force. Therefore, to stay in step with the increased power of the vital force and be slightly stronger than the power of the illness, the power of the next dose must also be slightly increased.[110]

After thirty years of using centesimal potencies, the eminent practitioner Dr. James Tyler Kent,[111] offers these centesimal potency guidelines:

- After selecting the proper remedy, it is of prime importance to give it in the proper dose, not to repeat it too frequently and not to change the remedy too soon.
- Too high a potency gives unnecessary aggravation and then will not perform the best curative action.
- The ideal response is the one that gives no aggravation but amelioration. We do not seek to produce an aggravation that is not the best, not the longest curative effect.
- It is unsafe for the beginner to indulge the desire to repeat the remedy.
- The greatest mischief may come from repeating the remedy when a positive effect has been obtained.
- Never repeat the dose or change the remedy when the patient is improving.
- Repetition of the dose to intensify the action of the remedy must not be considered as the rule.
- Never change a remedy unless the changed symptoms call for another remedy.
- The indiscriminate use of only one potency is very likely to bring reproach upon our art. From the thirtieth to the millionth, they all have their place.

---

[110] Dr. S. Hahnemann, *The Organon of Medicine*, Sixth edition, §247 and f/n 133

[111] Dr. J.T. Kent, *Lectures on Homœopathic Philosophy*, and *Kent's New Remedies, Clinical Cases, Lesser Writings, Aphorisms and Precepts*, compiled by Dr. W.W. Sherwood.

- We might well begin with Hahnemann's statement that the 30c is low enough or strong enough to start with. For many years I have found it strong enough to begin with.

- Some patients are very sensitive to the highest potencies and are cured mildly and permanently with 200c or 1M. There are other individuals who are torn to pieces by the highest potencies.

- Sometimes very sensitive patients will do well on a high potency, if a lower one has prepared them for it. I have frequently seen patients recover from their symptoms for a while under the 1M and then the remedy would cease to act. The 10M would then produce a very beneficial effect and make the cure permanent.

- No single potency is equal to the demands made upon it by the diseases of different individuals. Then the nature of the disease makes a difference; patients who have heart disease, or who are suffering from tuberculosis are apt to have their sufferings increased and the end hastened by the highest potencies; they do better under the 30c and 200c.

- The prolonged action is sometimes necessary in very chronic deep-seated diseases. A few months would exhaust the action of any drug if only one potency were used. Any potency, no matter what it is, high or low, will cease to act after a time. That shows at once the usefulness of knowing about more than one single potency of a medicine.

- I have been told by many homœopathic physicians that they have used the 3c, 6c, 12c, and obtained a fair result and then it ceased to act at all. Such prescribers have no range of potency and they fail to make a complete cure.

- From the crude to 10M there is a range of degrees in the ordinary person. You can repeat the series, beginning with the lower potencies and do good work. The patient will recognise these series.

- From experience, I am led to use a series (of ascending potencies) from 1M to DM.
- You encourage the patient to become oversensitive by using the highest potencies, instead of going low to begin (the series) again.
- It's a mistake to mix degrees and makes (manufacturers).
- If one has been started, stick to the same series and same scale.

6

Effective Patient Monitoring

Until a patient ingests a homœopathic medicine, if and exactly how their vital force will respond is unknown, which is why the homœopathic patient progress consultation is both thrilling and demanding. Practitioners pivot on the edge of jeopardising patient recovery, and the potential for misunderstanding vital force responses looms large. Perceiving the changed state of the vital force—or not—in response to the medicine, and knowing what to do next to assist it towards completion of cure, is often more challenging and complicated than making the first, or previous, prescription and may explain why many practitioners elect not to schedule progress examinations and instead leave patients or their guardians to judge whether or not they should report any changes. It is hoped such a relaxed strategy is not adopted during acute states or where the patients's mental state prevents the possibility of making such a judgement.

In the progress examination, as is necessary during the illness history taking phase, successful homœopathic patient monitoring requires practitioner intelligence, attentive listening, endless patience, rigorous observation, deep concentration and meticulous record keeping. A lot of information must be gathered to answer many questions, including:

- What happened after the prescribed remedy and dose was taken and what evidence supports that fact?
- Has the remedy affected the vital force at all? If not, why not?
- Has the remedy affected the vital force curatively or non-curatively?
- Is the vital force continuing to respond?
- Has the vital force stopped responding?
- What should I do next and why?
- How long should I watch and wait before acting?
- Exactly what am I waiting for?
- What is the next action to take and why?
- Is another dose of the same medicine required?
- Should the same or a different dose be administered?
- Is a different remedy required?
- Why did that response occur, and what evidence supports that fact?
- Has the state of the patient's vital force changed, and what evidence supports that fact?
- If the patient's state has changed, in what way has it changed and what evidence supports that fact?
- Has the patient's state become weaker, stronger, to what degree and what evidence supports that fact?
- Have the characteristic, distinguishing, individualising symptoms of the patient changed, and what evidence supports the fact those changes have occurred?
- Have the common symptoms of the illness changed, how and what does that indicate?
- What demonstrable evidence indicates that the patient is truly better, unchanged or worse?
- Does the response of the patient's vital force indicate the correct Direction of Cure?
- How do I know whether the response indicates the remedy that was selected was only partially accurate, versus completely accurate?

- Does the response of the vital force indicate cure or palliation (make a disease or its symptoms less severe or unpleasant without removing the cause)?

No matter how hard we try to avoid making mistakes, when faced with the complex, individual nature of each patient's vital force, all kinds of errors are possible for all manner of reasons. Recognising that an error has been made is the first step to correcting it.

To avoid confusion and to keep the patient moving smoothly along the path the recovery, unparalleled mental acuity; reliance upon intelligent, logical, well-reasoned thinking; a self-critical attitude and the highest degree of diligence, is required. To free ourselves from hopes, fears, presuppositions and biases towards and against possible results, we must continuously strive to demonstrate that peculiar objective state Hahnemann terms 'the unprejudiced observer'. It is essential to think systematically towards clarity.

Anyone using homœopathic medicines should be aware of when it is wise and beneficial to repeat a dose. Many consumers of homœopathy are unaware of the fact that Hahnemann discovered that all medicines have the power to alter the state of health always and unconditionally. And it is important not to forget that—in Hahnemann's original experiments—to understand the effects of medicines on healthy human beings, medicinal doses were administered twice daily specifically to induce symptoms. The results of these experiments proved that a homœopathic medicine taken repeatedly in the same unmodified dose does produce symptoms. The instruction for the centesimal potency: 'take one dose every two or three hours' without regard to whether there is improvement or worsening of symptoms, inappropriately applies mainstream medical practice protocols and ignores the fact that to achieve cure using homœopathy, only a minimal dose is required. In response to the correctly selected medicine and dose, the vital force responds curatively to the first dose and the symptoms being treated begin to disappear. However, because the medicine taken has the power to induce similar symptoms to those experienced, continuing to dose repeatedly several times daily, for a week, month or more, hinders the vital force instead of helping it. The vital force becomes extremely irritated by the repetition and bodily resistance to the medicine ensues. The initial curative response is interrupted. After a short relief of the original symptoms following the first dose, they return, only this time they are greatly intensified. Additionally, since each substance has the power to produce hundreds of symptoms (e.g. Calcarea Carbonica, has been proven to induce sixteen hundred and thirty individual symptoms), any number of different symptoms to those prescribed in the initial illness may appear alongside them. When these new symptoms appear, it is natural to think—incorrectly—that the patient is worse and another illness has erupted, meaning a different medicine is required. However, the most useful and safest thing to do is instruct the patient to *stop* taking that medicine and leave the vital force alone, without medicine, to allow the similar and different symptoms it induced to disappear on their own. This recovery from over-treatment is the best outcome, but cannot be guaranteed. It will only happen where the medicine selected was suitable, the dose was a moderate one and there is sufficient strength of vital force still prevailing in the patient.

Another significant obstacle to effective homœopathy is the casual approach of some prescribers and reluctance of some patients to report changes. Some prescribers only want to administer medicines and prefer not to monitor patient response. Some patients think if they report a worsening of their condition the practitioner will believe that they're being a nuisance, complaining or making trouble, and will drop them. So, they keep silent, muddle through severe, intensified suffering or relapse alone without help.

Persuading patients to report all changes—major or minor, good or bad—is a recurring feature of homœopathic patient education. In my own practice, I have to keep reminding my clients that the homœopathic healing process is a fifty-fifty patient–practitioner collaborative effort, and to restore full health, I need their help as much they need mine. My expertise lies in medicine and dose selection. Their expertise lies in describing what's going on in their body and mind. I'm powerless to keep them on the path to recovery if they don't tell me what's going on, especially when they don't feel well.

The other reason patients keep silent is because they believe a myth that is woven into the fabric of homœopathy: 'symptoms must always get worse before they get better'. Hahnemann explodes that myth. If symptoms *do* worsen and cure *is* taking place, the intensification of symptoms is very brief and always swiftly followed by significant improvement. Where the worsened state lingers, something has definitely gone wrong. Either the medicine or potency was incorrectly selected.[112] Dr. Kent also points out you will find very satisfactory cures, where the administration of the remedy is followed by no aggravation whatever. If there is no aggravation and recovery of the patient, the potency just exactly fitted the case.[113]

It is important to ensure no harm comes to patients. To do this, homœopathic practitioners have a duty to monitor patient responses to medicines diligently. To re-examine patients for more than anecdotal evidence and to check for clear signs of a directional shift of symptoms that indicate the vital force is responding—whether curatively or non-curatively.

To accurately determine whether or not the patient is moving in the natural curative direction, patient progress information received is compared to information already documented in:

- Original illness Totality of Characteristic Individualising Symptoms hierarchy (or 'The Working')
- Birth to Present Timeline that reflects the order in which each symptom, condition first appeared

Where a prescriber has not created such documents, effective patient progress assessment is impossible.

Hahnemann offers the most reliable, consistent advice concerning how to determine if, how, in what sphere of the body and to what degree the individual's vital force was or was not affected by a dose of homœopathic medicine, and whether the patient's vital force continues to respond or has stopped responding.

Gentle health restoration happens when the practitioner:

- Understands if and how the individual's vital force has been affected by a medicine

---

[112] Dr. S. Hahnemann, *The Organon of Medicine*, §161

[113] Dr. J. T. Kent, *Lectures on Homœopathic Philosophy*

- Knows how to keep dose administration in step with recovery pace of the vital force
- Observes the patient carefully at certain intervals after each dose of medicine and before further treatment for any symptom changes that may occur
- Notes and intelligently interprets all changes experienced

It is during the first and all subsequent patient progress review consultations that the patient and practitioner arrive at a crossroad. The direction in which symptoms and patient move, towards or away from cure, depend on the quality of information gathered during this review.

Formulating and posing high-quality questions elicits high-quality information. Promptly weighing all the pros and cons is a great challenge. Where there is the slightest doubt about what a particular piece of information means or what action to take and why, expert practitioners take an extra moment to pause and think a little longer to obtain clarity before taking any action. In my own practice, I tell patients 'I'm going to be silent for a few seconds while I think what I am going to do and why. Then I'll explain my thought process and decisions.' Given a particular complexity, if the required action involves an element of risk (e.g. it is an action the practitioner has never taken before), it is always wise and respectful to be up front, discuss the nature and degree of the risk with the patient and seek their consent *before* giving a risky instruction. That way the patient shares in the decision that affects their health and feels respected.

The purpose of examining and evaluating the individual's general and particular improvement or decline in response to the medicine is to understand what and where the changes have occurred, and what the degree and nature of these changes are. As practitioners, we seek to discern whether the individual's vital force is able or unable to respond to the medicine. We need to know whether the remedy taken penetrated deeply into the body, affected the whole of the person and had a lasting effect, or acted superficially on part of the person and was capable of only temporary effect.

As well as certain review questions, other essential instruments of inquiry that make the difference between practitioner clarity and confusion are:

- Careful observation
- Attentive listening
- Logical examination based on knowledge of the fixed principles
- Exceptional critical thinking skills

Throughout the homœopathic self-healing process, patient education is crucial. This is especially the case with regard to prohibiting self-medication with over-the-counter medicines—especially homœopathic medicines. The disruptive influence of self-medication must be addressed at the outset of treatment and, where possible, eliminated. It's a difficult topic to broach because patients think self-medicating is part of taking charge of their health. They are unaware that the body is *always, unconditionally altered by all medicines* and seldom consider how different combinations of medicines might harm the body. For recovery to be smooth, they also need to know that once treatment has begun, any unauthorised self-medication with homœopathic medicines tends to delay rapid gentle recovery. The curative effects of well-chosen prescriptions may be interrupted indefinitely, and uncertainty about which medicine caused which response, may cause practitioner confusion and commission of serious case management errors. Therefore, it is reasonable to request an undertaking from patients not self-prescribe without practitioner consent. In order to remind patients of their commitment, it is wise to begin each progress report with the question: *what medicines have you taken since our last consultation?*

From the first consultation onwards, it is vital to educate patients and their guardians that, in homœopathy, the slightest change of state might signal that the vital force has been strongly influenced by the homœopathic remedy. Therefore, any changes—whether major or minor; subtle or dramatic; mental, emotional and physical shifts—*must* be reported to the practitioner for evaluation. For this to happen, patients need to be firmly told that practitioners of homœopathy welcome updates from patients between progress reports.

The proper interval between each patient progress review varies according to whether treatment is for longstanding or sudden-onset, acute, emergency illnesses.

For longstanding illness, progress reviews are best conducted at four- to five-week intervals. Patients are invited to report in between if they require clarification about what is happening to them. As the patient improves and moves towards complete health restoration, the intervals between reviews extend, for example from once every month for three months, to once every other month and so on.

In chronic illness treatment using the LM/Q[114] potency scale, correct intervals between reports begin with very brief five to seven-day interval reports plus an extensive monthly report. Once the patient is familiar with the dosing method, the five to seven-day reports stop and only monthly reports are required. If the patient experiences any changes other than improvement, it is their duty to report that change, before the scheduled review if necessary. Such changes indicate a minor adjustment to the dosing regimen may be required.

For sudden-onset, severe illness, progress reviews are conducted at five-, ten-, fifteen-, thirty- and sixty-minute intervals. Then, as the patient improves, the intervals extend to once every two hours, etc. until the excruciating headache and nausea, or the bruised swollen eye disappears. The severity of an illness dictates the exact interval of time between reports. For example, loss of body fluids (haemorrhage, diarrhoea, vomiting and high fevers or collapse) demand much shorter intervals than the slightly longer intervals needed for debilitating head pain.

Acute-state, urgent-need conditions typically come on rapidly and forcefully. They might indicate the vital force is up and running and able to swiftly resolve what may be a life-threatening circumstance without help. Or they could suggest that the vital force is on the verge of being completely overwhelmed. To keep pace with the volatile vital force, urgent care progress report intervals must err on the side of caution and be scheduled very frequently: five or ten minutes rather than hours.

Accurate progress report information must overcome several common obstacles.

---

[114] See Chapter 11, LM Potency Response Analysis

> In deciding the question whether the remedy has acted or not, we must be careful not to be misled by the opinions or prejudices of the patient or his attendants. Some patients, having all their interest and attention centred upon some particular symptom, which they regard as all-important, will assert that there has been no change; that they are no better, or even worse than they were before they took the remedy. These statements should be received with great caution and we should proceed to go over the symptom-record item by item with care. We need not antagonize the patient by gruffly asserting that he must be mistaken, but may express our regret or sympathy and then quietly question him as to each particular symptom. We will frequently find that the patient has really improved in many important respects, although the pet symptom (often constipation) is yet unchanged.[115]

> We have in the symptoms that which we can rely upon... The symptoms themselves must be corroborated. The patient's opinion must be corroborated by the symptoms. The symptoms do corroborate what the patient says in many instances, but the symptoms are the physician's most satisfactory evidence.[116]

Another obstacle is practitioner bias towards a particular outcome. This stems from practitioner fear of failure and desperation for a curative response. The bias is displayed in leading questions posed by the practitioner; for example, 'that heart fluttering you had, there isn't any chest pain with it, right?' In order to overcome that obstacle, open-ended questions must be formulated and posed and patients and guardians invited to think deeply before they answer; for example, 'Tell me everything about how the heart is now.'

Practitioner complacency regarding patient responses such as: 'I feel great; I'm fine; I'm OK; I am completely healed!' is yet another obstacle. The human condition being what it is, the natural desire to be successful excites the temptation for practitioners to accept such answers at face value without verifying the truth. To accept such vague answers as definitive proof of cure strengthens the claims of those who oppose homœopathy and believe that patient responses to homœopathic medicines are merely anecdotal.

Verification of the truth is also important when patient reports are at the other extreme and, horror of horrors, the practitioner is told

---

[115] Dr. S. Close, *The Genius of Homœopathy*

[116] Dr. J.T. Kent, *Lectures on Homœopathic Philosophy*

'nothing happened, everything is the same'; 'I'm in a very bad way'; 'my baby looks terrible'; 'my dog is still scratching', etc. Either way, we must maintain our concentration and composure, and examine patient remarks carefully and thoroughly, complete the progress report and gain clarity concerning decisions and actions to be taken. A useful way to clarify vague reports is to invite the patient to: 'say more about' or 'give me an example of the way you feel fine, in a bad way', etc.

Patient progress examination for urgent and longstanding illness is much more structured than the free-flowing-history taking inquiry. However, it must be just as thorough. For consistency, the patient's state after the remedy is taken *is always* compared to the patient's original symptom totality portrait, i.e. the individualising features, sensations, modifying conditions, etc., that was reported and recorded at the history intake *before* the remedy was taken.

For example, a typical urgent care symptom totality portrait might look like this:

Patient state *before* the remedy is administered:
General Mental, Emotional Disposition:
- Desires to be carried
- Averse to being left alone

General Physical Disposition:
- Person and symptoms worse in the evening

Particulars (in order of first appearance):
- Nose: running, worse evening
- Nose: running, with cough
- Cough: mucous in chest
- Face: discolouration red during cough

Patient state reported *after* taking the remedy:
General Mental, Emotional Disposition:
- Desire to be carried disappears
- Aversion to being left alone disappears

General Physical Disposition:
- Worsening of symptoms in the evening disappears

Particulars (in order of first appearance):

- Nose: running much less and no worse during evening
- Nose: running with cough is fifty to sixty percent improved
- Cough: there is no mucous in chest
- Face: no red discolouration during cough because the cough is much improved

In reviewing chronic illness progress, the instrument of comparison is The Working: the original illness Totality of Characteristic Individualising Symptoms (TCIS) document. It allows easy, accurate assessment of how and in what way patient and symptoms improve, worsen or remain unchanged. The TCIS will be larger in chronic-illness monitoring than in the acute state, emergency-care monitoring. Using the TCIS for comparison is particularly helpful for patients trying to remember how they felt before taking the remedy. They are unskilled in the art of homœopathic medical observation and unused to paying attention to any changes. If something has been rumbling on for a while and become part of their life, they often consider it unworthy of comment. The TCIS allows them to review exactly how they felt before they took the remedy. Very often, once a longstanding symptom disappears, patients tend to forget about it and fail to report changes in that symptom. Alternatively, in describing something considered to be completely new, they discover that it is a reappearance of an old forgotten symptom, perhaps returning in a slightly or dramatically altered form.

The individual's vital force, when responding to a remedy, issues a 'report card' concerning the practitioner's work.

The accuracy or inaccuracy of the practitioner's medicine and dose selection influences how the vital force is affected. If the vital force is strengthened sufficiently to overwhelm the disturbance, original symptoms change for the better, subside and disappear, and complete restoration of health occurs, then the patient feels terrific. If the remedy and dose affect the vital force to some degree but not completely, some symptoms will disappear then reappear and the patient feels somewhat improved. When the remedy and dose selection does not affect the vital force at all then the illness continues unabated, original symptoms remain unchanged or perhaps intensify, new symptoms appear and the patient feels worse. There are, of course, many variations of those results.

To ensure essential progress assessment information is gathered, a list of relevant questions should be prepared. Having done that, don't just go through each question and tick it off as done. Patients know when someone is paying attention to them or not. Slow down. Think carefully about its relevance before posing each question. Allow patients enough time to think deeply before they answer. Listen carefully to each answer before asking the next question. Make sure each answer offers useful information.

To ensure no stone is left unturned, check through the TCIS carefully so that the progress examination compares the status of all symptoms experienced, reported and documented before the remedy was taken.

Each change experienced indicates whether the vital force is or is not strengthening or weakening, is or is not moving in the curative direction.

To obtain high-quality information, it is necessary to formulate and pose high-quality, open questions. The list below will provide the high-quality progress-assessment information needed. Due to the individuality of each person and illness it might need to be extended. I have provided reasons for each question posed.

1. What medicines have you taken since we last consulted?

Answers to this question will reveal patient inadvertent or deliberate self-medication and allow the practitioner to consider any obstacle to recovery it might present and strategies for overcoming that obstacle.

2. Describe what happened after you took the remedy; how you feel generally overall since you took it.

Answers to this question reveal whether the vital force was affected by the medicine or not, whether it has been negatively or positively affected and how.

3. Describe exactly how the original symptoms that bothered you have changed for better, worse or remained unchanged.

The answer to this question usually provides information concerning changes to many of the original symptoms and conditions experienced, as opposed to information about just the chief complaint.

It has the potential to reveal dramatic as well as subtle and almost imperceptible shifts that might have occurred at some level in one direction or another. To ensure we receive information about the symptom totality, it is necessary to review each symptom one by one, asking: how is this or that symptom?

Degrees of change experienced after taking a remedy indicate improvement or worsening of symptoms. The scale 0–10 (zero to ten) is a useful device to measure improvement or worsening of each symptom. Here's an example of how it might be used:

4. For the sake of argument, on the scale 0–10, if ten out of ten was awarded for awfulness of your symptoms before you took the remedy, how many marks out of ten would you give the awfulness of that symptom, condition now? (Using the symptom image totality, mention each symptom, sensation for separate valuation).

As long as the patient is always reminded that zero means none and ten means excruciatingly intolerable, this 0–10, zero to ten, scale works especially well for pain symptoms. Patients who suffer pain for many years become inured to it and may not notice a slight change of degree in pain until questioned directly.

5. What significant changes have occurred regarding domestic or work circumstances?

The answer to this question provides information regarding external changes that may have occurred since the remedy was taken and might impinge on the patient's health. The answer also has the potential to reveal whether a patient is able to adapt appropriately and successfully to different life changes or not.

If it is clear from information received that absolutely nothing at all has changed on any level, ask:

6. Tell me about everything significant that happened since you took the remedy and how you were affected. Take a moment to think about your answer.

This answer may reveal a circumstance that interrupted a short-lived curative response. For example, the day after taking the remedy, the patient receives bad news, has a tooth root canal, has a car crash, or experiences some other trauma, injury or great shock to the body. This would be understood to be a 'proximate' cause. The answer may also elicit the existence of a new maintaining cause such as the illness or loss of a family member, or a job loss, and the patient had considered this to be unimportant or was too embarrassed to report. Such profound changes often disturb patients deeply enough to awaken a slumbering latent inherent predisposition to illness, resulting in severe imbalance at the core of the person. To understand the reason for the non-curative response, it is extremely important to know the difference between root (predisposition) and proximate (injury) causes, otherwise we risk erroneously changing a well-indicated medicine and spoiling and excellent prescription.

It is essential to investigate possible changes that may have occurred in a patient's faculty of reasoning **or emotional** state. To do so effectively requires understanding that, when ill, the ability to concentrate is often affected. Longer questions are more difficult to answer clearly. Individuals often forget what was asked at the beginning of the question and only recall the last part, so they only answer the last part and leave the other part(s) unanswered. Consequently, unless we are listening attentively and notice information gaps, incomplete information is received and wrong decisions are made. Shorter questions better. A different question should be asked about each function i.e. one that relates to reasoning, one that relates to comprehension/understanding, and one that relates to the emotional sphere. To ensure clarity always ask for examples. Questions such as these work well.

7. Describe changes experienced in your feelings.

8. Describe changes experienced in how you express your emotions.

9. Described changes experienced in your worries.

10. Describe changes experienced in your cravings, longings.

11. Describe changes in your aversions.

12. Describe changes in your ability to think and reason.

13. Describe changes in your concentration, focus.

14. Describe changes in your ability remember things.

15. Describe changes experienced in your motivation.

As well as changes in motivational, intellectual and emotional spheres that may have occurred, we also need to know the following: whether there are any changes in the way the patient survives and adjusts to stresses; how they are affected by worry; whether old constraining emotions burdening the vital force before treatment have lifted or been released; whether a previous tendency to suppress feelings due fear of what might happen if they were to express them, continues or has ceased.

Examples include: in response to the first or previous medicine, we may observe a withdrawn, shut-down person before taking the medicine become lively, active and expressive afterwards. A self-conscious patient who, before the remedy always only wept alone, after the remedy weeps openly in front of others without being bothered by it at all. Or a person who is sorrowful and suicidal before a remedy is taken becomes lighthearted, happier, smiling and laughing, optimistic and highly motivated afterwards. These examples indicate improvements.

However, were we to receive information that, without provocation of any kind, a reserved person becomes more reserved; a happy person becomes sad and depressed, an outgoing person becomes withdrawn, etc., the individual's state of mind is considered to have worsened. To confirm without a doubt the truth of such information, asking Question 6 again and listening to the answer usually works well. Another way to corroborate the regression is to immediately check back through the original record. This should confirm or deny that the current symptoms are not a reappearance of an old state of mind that had been temporarily relieved or suppressed by mainstream medication or other means in the past and had not been reported earlier. If there is no record of the state in the original illness history and there is no apparent cause for the downward shift, it would be useful to ask:

16. When in your life have you experienced these feelings or something like them before?

The answer to this question tends to reveal the return of an old state that has been forgotten and not reported at history-taking. This return would indicate that the remedy had been well-chosen. The remedy has assisted the vital force in excavating an old symptom, bringing it up to the surface for permanent resolution. Chapter 9 offers information about actions to take when patients experience deterioration in their mental and emotional state after taking centesimal potency doses. Chapter 11 offers the same information after patients receive LM/Q potency doses.

Sleep is the bridge between the active and resting mind. To assess sleep pattern changes, the next question is useful:

17. Compared to before you took the remedy, describe the changes you have experienced regarding your sleep pattern and how you feel when you wake up.

Ideally sleep satisfies our need for rest; we awake refreshed ready and eager to start each day's activities. Experience indicates that the vital force often uses the dreaming process to vent disturbances at the innermost without causing excessive disruption elsewhere in the organism. This is especially true of dreams in which previously unresolved matters are resolved. Therefore, the answer to this question is important because it may also reveal aspects of the patient's intellectual emotional experience, which is a useful indication of what is going on at the deepest core of the patient.

If sexual sphere symptoms were part of the original symptom totality, ask:

18. What changes have you experienced in the sexual sphere?

The next question concerns the individual's physical energy.

19. Overall, how has your energy vitality been affected since you took the remedy? Describe the level on which the energy changes have taken place and the degree of change experienced.

In health, we have enough energy to undertake all activities plus some held in reserve for emergency situations requiring masses of energy for a short time, e.g. the survival of a disaster.

This answer to this question reveals whether there has been an increase or loss of physical energy and to what degree this has happened, and offers important information about the strength or weakness of the patient's vital force. To gain clarity, don't settle for vague information. Request specific examples to illustrate energy level changes. For comparison, the measurement 0–10 is useful. In this case, zero equals no energy and ten equals lots of energy. It is crucial that practitioners to know that patients often misunderstand this energy-level question. Patients tend to think they are being measured against other people's energy levels, rather than their own. They need to be reminded that it is their own energy and view of it that is used for assessment. I had one patient who consistently reported his energy level never went higher than 2/10. Yet his mental and physical symptoms had dramatically improved. He was back at the gym and taking the dog for lengthy walks. When I said the low energy reported didn't make sense, given the improvements in activity, the patient replied: 'Oh Joe Bloggs next door is far more energetic than I am, he's definitely a 10 out of 10, I'm nothing like that. Compared to him I'm 2 out of 10.' Once I had reminded the patient exactly who was being measured, it turned out he felt he had 60% more energy after the remedy than before. But Joe Bloggs still had more!

20. Describe any changes in previous patterns, habits, you have experienced regarding how you are affected by: e.g. changes in temperature, the weather, time of the month, season of the year or food.

This question is posed to reveal any changes that relate to the patient as a whole. For example, before the remedy, the patient was adversely affected by weather changes that induced terrible headaches. After the remedy, the patient experiences weather changes completely free of headaches. Since it is another long question, in order to overcome the loss of concentration obstacle, ask the same question separately for each of the five topics mentioned.

21. (For females): How were you before, during and after your last menstrual flow?

This is an extremely important question to ask. The answer concerns a discharge from the inside of the organism. In homœopathy all discharges from any orifice are extremely significant. They indicate the innermost condition of the individual's vital force. Therefore, considerable attention must always be paid to discharges and related changes.

Also, the menstrual cycle is an integral part of each female. Therefore, information concerning unexpected absence of, and changes in the menstrual cycle or blood flow, including reappearance of menstrual flow after having ceased during menopause, is very useful in determining improvement or worsening of illness at the interior of the person. Depending on the individual, changes related to the physical, mental and emotional spheres might occur around the menstrual blood flow. The answer to this question offers great insight into what is happening to the female as a whole since the remedy was taken.

(For post-menopausal females): *Although the discharge of blood aspect of the menstrual cycle has ceased, the hormone cycle continues. Have you noticed any changes around the time when you used to bleed?*

22. Describe any new symptoms that you have never experienced before in your life.

The answer to this question may be especially significant. Appearance of truly new, never-experienced-before symptoms and conditions always worry patients and practitioners equally. In longstanding illnesses, very often a symptom considered by a patient to be new is truthfully not new at all. It could be the reappearance of an old symptom in a slightly modified form, an old symptom that was forgotten because it disappeared long ago, or it is a symptom that the patient has become used to over time. They consider it to be 'new' because increased intensity of the symptom has drawn the patient's attention to it and perhaps induced anxiety about it. To confirm the 'new' symptoms mentioned by the patient are truly new (compared to being old ones in a new guise) take a moment to scan the history of illness timeline thoroughly. See Chapter 10 Non-Curative Response Analysis and Chapter 11 LM/Q Potency Response Analysis for a detailed discussion of the Appearance of New Symptoms and appropriate actions to be taken.

It is very unwise to finish the progress report interview without the certainty that you fully understand everything about all the changes that have or have not occurred, and you have noted prominent as well as subtle stabilisation, destabilisation, improvement or worsening of the patient's state in its entirety. Responsibility for clarity belongs the practitioner. If there is in any doubt about the information offered in answer to a question, always ask the patient to elaborate. Ask something along the lines of: 'Please explain in more detail what you mean by....'

While the patient delivers their progress report, we are determined not to miss anything; to know if the vital force was affected by the remedy and dose taken, whether our aim was true and we hit the bullseye or if we fell short of the target.

After a prescription has been made, the physician begins to make observations. The whole future of the patient may depend upon the conclusions that the physician arrives at from these observations, for his action depends very much upon his observations, and upon his action depends the good of the patient. If he is not conversant with the import of what he sees, he will undertake to do wrong things, he will make wrong prescriptions, and he will change his medicines and do things to the detriment of the patient.[117]

Use this checklist to ensure the progress examination provides enough accurate information for analysis.

- Always have the patient's files in front of you.
- Always use the original symptom totality as the instrument of comparison.
- Always know what information you seek and why you are posing a particular question.
- Always formulate open questions.
- Always listen attentively to ensure the answer given relates to the question asked.
- Always check the detail of what the patient reports.
- Always seek corroboration of information.
- Always ask for concrete examples of changes.
- Never accept vague answers.
- If confused by an answer, always ask the patient or guardian to elaborate until the information is clearly understood.
- When patients report 'I am all better' or 'nothing happened,' continue the review to confirm or deny the truth of that statement.
- Never end the progress report without being confident that all necessary and relevant information has been gathered. If there are gaps in your understanding, ask (more) open-ended questions to gain further clarity.
- Always ensure the information received enables you to decide what action to take next and why.

---

[117] Dr. J.T. Kent, *Lectures on Homœopathic Philosophy*

Having examined the patient to discover whether or not the vital force responded to the medicine, next we have to understand what that response indicates. There are three parts to that thought process. The first part (Chapter 7) involves understanding what to look for at the progress report so that the information received is considered in the proper context and response misinterpretation is minimised. The second part (Chapter 8) discusses the purpose of watchful waiting. The third part (Chapters 9, 10 and 11) involves evaluating the responses and deciding what to do next and why

7

How to Avoid Misinterpreting Responses

Due to the highly refined, delicate nature of the vital force, it takes minimal misinterpretation of a patient's progress report to interrupt a curative response and spoil the effect of an excellent prescription.

> I have always regretted and never forgotten a spoilt Lachesis case—spoilt for want of [then] knowledge. It was a huge cavity in a woman's calf; one of those big excavated ulcers one used to see so often in student days. Lachesis was her remedy and was prescribed. The second time she appeared, there was most amazing healing in the ulcer. Instead of waiting to let the vital reaction carry on towards cure, it was interrupted by repetition of the remedy. When she came again it was much worse, and then she came no more. It was a tragedy. 'My people perish for lack of knowledge.' Work is not always easy, but spoiling good work is easy and deplorable. When things are going well, past all expectation, let them get on with it. Solomon says, 'there is a time for everything' but the time of rapid extraordinary improvement is not the time to butt in.[118]

To avoid confusion and keep the patient moving smoothly along the path of recovery, unparalleled practitioner mental acuity and reliance upon intelligent, logical, well-reasoned thinking is required. We put aside our innate love of ease, engage the intellect, avoid haste, and

---

[118] Dr. J.T. Kent, *Lectures on Homœopathic Materia Medica*

move thoughtfully, systematically towards clarity. In that way, clinical errors are reduced, rapidly identified and corrected.

Given the uniqueness of each state of suffering experienced, each individual's vital force of nature has its own unique curative momentum. It is foolhardy for patients and practitioners to expect a disorganised, weakened vital force to respond within a precise predetermined period, and also to think that the vital force enjoys being hurried along the road to recovery. It doesn't. It prefers gentle treatment, time to regroup and time to redirect its recovery force.

> A remedy shows its action, 1) by producing new symptoms; 2) by the disappearance of symptoms; 3) by the increase or aggravation of symptoms; 4) by the amelioration of symptoms; 5) by a change in the order and direction of symptoms.[119]

To accurately determine whether or not the patient is moving in the orderly natural direction of cure, once again the instruments for comparison are: (a) original illness characteristic individualising symptom totality, and (b) chronological birth to present symptom timeline that reflects the order in which each symptom or condition first appeared. Such detailed records are of particular importance when assisting medically mismanaged patients because these patients' weary vital force often opts for an indirect route to recovery.

Every aspect of the patient's progress report must be meticulously examined regarding the degree of symptom intensity change, whether it increases, decreases or doesn't change. Are the symptoms indicating the patient is moving in the curative inward-to-outward direction: from the mental plane to the physical plane, or non-curative outward to inward direction: from the physical plane to mental/emotional plane?

Factors affecting response pace include:
- The degree of vital force prevailing before a remedy was taken
- Prior treatment received
- Whether the remedy selected had the power to induce the greatest number of similar symptoms to the symptoms

---

[119] Dr. S. Close, *The Genius of Homœopathy*

experienced by the patient and was administered in the proper dose

- Curability potential of state
- Whether the state being treated is urgent care or longstanding

Typical response timeframes for urgent care states vary from within seconds to minutes. Recovery from longstanding illness usually begins within hours, days or a few weeks.

After ingesting the exactly correct homœopathic medicine and dose that hit the bull's eye dead centre, patients experience an immediate lasting improvement. Where the prescription was slightly off-centre, a fleeting, slight intensification of the original existing symptoms occurs, during which time, oddly, the patient feels much better overall. We may feel better immediately or after a short delay.

When the body is in recovery mode, the ideal curative order in which symptoms change is:

1. Most recent symptom(s) to appear are usually first to disappear.
2. First symptoms to appear are usually the last to disappear.
3. Symptoms move from most vital organ to least vital organ, and from the head to hands and feet.
4. The natural curative response of the vital force is always centrifugal. Symptoms move from within outwards.

We must distinguish between changes occurring within vital organs and changes in superficial tissues and non-vital organs. For example, organs related to the digestive tract are more vital to the preservation of life than fingernails. Depending on the strength or weakness of the patient's vital force, original symptoms of the disturbance move from the interior nucleus towards the exterior surface, of every part of the body. Often there is a discharge of some kind: e.g. tears, diarrhoea, vomit, increased urination, pus, perspiration; nasal, vaginal or urethral mucous; or the disorder is vented through a rash, pustules, vesicles, boils or warts on the skin.

Since the aim of the pure homœopathic healing art is the annihilation of the underlying causation(s) and central disturbance of the disease to complete restoration of health:

...We should know by the symptoms if the changes occurring are sufficiently interior... So that by the symptoms we can know whether the changes that are occurring are of sufficient depth, so that the patient may recover.[120]

For example, in a longstanding illness:

When old skin eruptions reappear, old ulcers break out again, old fistulae reopen, old discharges flow again, swollen tubercular glands become inflamed, break down and suppurate away; old joint pains return; the patient's heart, lung, kidney, liver, spleen or brain symptoms in the meantime *improving*, then we know that both remedy and dose were right and a true cure is in progress. But if we find superficial symptoms disappearing and vital organs showing signs of advancing disease, we know we have failed.[121]

Incurable diseases will very often be palliated by mild medicines that act only superficially, act upon the senses though the hidden and deep-seated trouble goes on and progresses and is sometimes made worse, yet the patient is made comfortable.[122]

Let's take an illness that came on suddenly where all the symptoms were extremely intense. First, the moderate fever with perspiration appeared (common symptom of many illnesses, less life-threatening), followed by nausea (more life-threatening), followed by vomiting and then bloody diarrhoea (loss of body fluids are the most life-threatening).

In recovery mode the vital force usually eliminates symptoms in reverse: first, the bloody diarrhoea and vomiting stops, then the nausea and finally the moderate fever which is the least life-threatening discomfort.

With a nosebleed, it starts as a trickle, gathers pace then gushes out the nose. After correct the remedy and dose, within seconds the gushing flow disappears *first*, the trickle flow reappears, then the trickle stops.

In understanding the meaning of symptom changes after the remedy is taken, it is necessary to pay attention to possible simple and complicated shifts in the underlying inherited predisposition(s) and the

---

[120] Dr. J. T. Kent, *Lectures on Homœopathic Philosophy*

[121] Dr. S. Close, *The Genius of Homœopathy*

[122] Dr. J. T. Kent, *Lectures on Homœopathic Philosophy*

exciting or maintaining causations. It may happen that an exciting cause (simple) becomes a maintaining cause (complicated). For example, the painful swollen ankle injury (exciting) persists or flares up repeatedly (maintaining). Or there's a shift in the activity of inherent predispositions to illness: before the remedy a predisposition was slumbering, dormant; after the remedy it is aroused and wreaks havoc, or vice versa. Very often, incurable diseases will be palliated by medicines that act only superficially, acting upon the senses, even though the hidden and more deep-seated trouble goes on and progresses. In this case, it is sometimes made worse, yet the patient is made comfortable.[123]

Up to now we've considered situations where the vital force was affected by a remedy and dose. But what if the patient's report indicates no change has occurred at any spirit, mind, body level? Such a lack of reaction indicates the remedy has not influenced the vital force at all.

If this occurs, hold your horses! Don't immediately jump to the conclusion that a different remedy or dose is needed to solve the problem. To avoid incurring a muddle, it is vital that we take the time to think clearly. We must ask ourselves why the chosen remedy didn't affect the vital force in any way shape or form. Until we understand what has happened, we cannot know with any certainty that changing the remedy is the correct action. We would only be guessing, speculating that the first prescription was an error.

We must discriminate between that which is reaction and that which calls for a remedy.[124]

It is common for the vital force not to react to a particular remedy if:

1. There has been an error in remedy selection due to an error in the symptom totality view
2. There has been an error in potency selection
3. A combination of both (1) and (2)
4. The vital force has been so severely weakened by prior long-continued medical mismanagement that its recovery power has

---

[123] Dr. J. T. Kent, *Lectures on Homœopathic Philosophy*

[124] Dr. J.T. Kent, *Lectures on Homœopathic Philosophy*

been almost obliterated and needs more time to marshal its limited resources

5. The recovery power of the vital force is severely curtailed by advanced pathology

6. Obstacles to cure exist; for example, maintaining causes, or concurrent use of other medicinal substances

To accurately decipher vital force responses to remedies, it is necessary to determine whether the prescription was effective and restored continuous permanent health, or ineffective and the symptoms have been a) forcibly removed usually through improper repetition of doses, or b) palliated: made less severe or more tolerable without removing the root cause.

Intelligent evaluation of the patient's response to the remedy will lead to one of the following decisions and actions:

- Before making a second prescription, wait watchfully for the proper length time to elapse for symptoms to disappear and recur with less intensity, or disappear or subside without recurring
- Decide to repeat the same remedy in the same potency
- Decide to repeat the same remedy in a modified ascending potency
- According to the LM/Q daily dosing regimen, stop or resume dosing (see Chapter 11)
- Decide to select a new remedy and dosing regimen

The next chapter discusses the important role played by knowledgeable, purposeful, *watchful* waiting.

8

Watchful Waiting

A conscientious homœopathic practitioner does nothing carelessly, and is not driven by impatience. Many a life is saved by watchful waiting that is always governed by knowledge and with a fixed purpose. Proficiency in homœopathy requires practitioners to shift their mindset away from thinking that waiting always implies inactivity. On the contrary, waiting watchfully during ongoing case management involves monitoring the patient frequently, carefully weighing the need for another dose against the need to watch and wait for the patient's vital force to direct us to the next action. We are not only waiting for something *to* happen; we are also waiting *while* something is happening.

> The inner nature of the disease appears to the physician through the symptoms, and it is like watching the hands on the clock. This watching and waiting and observing has to be done by the physician so that he may judge by the changes what to do, and what not to do. There is always an index that tells him what not to do ... if he is a sharp and vigilant observer he will see the index for every case.[125]

Here's an excellent example of knowledgeable, purposeful, watchful waiting in an urgent-care patient. Note that while waiting,

---

[125] Dr. J. T. Kent, *Lectures on Homœopathic Philosophy*

Dr. Kent is watching his patient very closely and thinking deeply about what he observes.

A beautiful daughter, aged four, in the midst of luxury and dignity, was sickened with diphtheria. The family doctor was allopathic and attended to the little one unto the threshold of eternity, when in spite of his logic and bitter vituperations against homœopaths as a class, it was considered wise to change. A strong lotion had been used in the throat until it was but a black cavern...when the writer visited what remained of this once beautiful tiny human form. The room was aired, the linen changed, the drugs removed; plenty of water ordered for the patient. The child was sick, the family doctor said it had diphtheria; the throat was black with effect of drug work. The nurse did not know where the membrane had begun to form, did not know the color of the membrane; she knew the child had been sick four days, and had passed urine, but no stool; was prostrated and sick. She did not know what hours of the day it was better or worse in appearance...The larynx appeared clear as there was no rough breathing, which was a wonder. At 12.00, midday, the first prescription was water containing Sac Lac[126] every hour, day and night. Evening found the throat cleared of its blackness; the face of the patient was pale, deathly; the child was prostrated; pulse 120; some fever; scanty urine. Sac Lac continued; next morning the membrane began reforming on the right side. Midday the membrane spread to the left side; child thirsty, and takes plenty of water, no food; urine almost gone. That evening the membrane is still spreading toward the left; 4.pm. Child very nervous, whined and screamed out; quieted later in the evening.

Thirty-two hours have passed since the writer took charge of this case and nature has expressed the symptoms that call for one remedy, which could not be guessed in the beginning. The right to left spreading of the membrane and the 4 p.m. aggravation of the general state of the patient, Lycopodium CM (Finke), one dose and Sac Lac. Up to then it would have been guess work, negligence and carelessness to make a prescription...Anything less than waiting and watching would have been a violation of a fundamental rule of homœopathy. That much time (waiting) was necessary to ascertain the symptoms in that particular case.

Every experienced physician must now and then receive a case from the hands of the old school or from some incompetent prescriber, and

---

[126] The non-medicinal, inert Sac Lac sugar milk agent mentioned here is NOT to be confused with the modern homœopathic medicine called Sac Lac.

these spoiled cases often die, before the symptoms come back to show what remedy should be administered. The case above is now in perfect health, having had but the one dose of the appropriate medicine.

The members of this family are now strong advocates of homœopathy, and feel that their little one was saved by its principle and law.[127]

Learning to wait watchfully is extremely difficult. It requires three things: wisdom, courage and patience.[128] The above case clearly demonstrates not only the importance of avoiding the 'more haste less speed' mistake, but also the need for accurate homœopathic information to be gleaned before the correct remedy may be selected and administered in the proper dose at proper intervals. On many occasions, homœopathic waiting with purpose reduces suffering and hastens cure. Commonsense must be applied to each situation. Watchful purposeful waiting must never endanger life.

Success or failure in homœopathy depends on individual practitioner knowledge, intelligence and how well they understand and skilfully apply the rules of homœopathic *watchful* waiting.

I presume that most prescribers will say: 'We have often acted too soon, but never waited too long.' Many physicians fail because of not waiting, and the waiting must be governed by knowledge ... To know that this waiting is right is quite different from waiting without a fixed purpose.[129]

Timing of each dose is critical to cure. Waiting time without medicine varies. It is dictated by the strength of the vital force that prevails within each patient and whether suffering is intense, dangerous or longstanding. Accordingly, the waiting period before

---

[127] *Kent's New Remedies, Clinical Cases, Lesser Writings, Aphorisms and Precepts,* compiled by Dr. W. W. Sherwood

[128] Dr. S. Close, *The Genius of Homœopathy*

[129] *Kent's New Remedies, Clinical Cases, Lesser Writings, Aphorisms and Precepts,* compiled by Dr. W.W. Sherwood

acting might be seconds, minutes or hours; or days, weeks or months.

Beware! Nothing about the response of the vital force can be predicted with certainty. Don't be fooled into acting without the vital force signalling it either needs to be left alone, or it needs help. Conversely, don't be lulled into complacency and wait too long. To avoid missing the moment that the patient's vital force needs more help, homœopathic observation and progress assessment intervals should match the pace of the vital force, which is determined by the disappearance, reappearance and directional shift of symptoms. Waiting watchfully with a fixed purpose will be harder for some patients and practitioners than others.

> The doctor watches the improvement of the patient and the corresponding disappearance of the symptoms under [the influence of] the first prescription, and when the case comes to a standstill he is uneasy, and with increasing fidgetiness he awaits the coming indication for the next dose.

> This fidgetiness, which comes from a lack of knowledge, unfits the physician as an observer and judge of symptoms; hence we see the doctor usually failing to cure his own children. He cannot wait and reason clearly over the returning symptoms.[130]

Calmly watching and waiting for the individual's vital force to respond naturally, to move at its own pace, requires both the patient and practitioner to think beyond the need to automatically intervene with medication if symptoms worsen. Continuous, permanent restoration of health using homœopathy demands courage and perseverance from both patient and practitioner.

There is much wisdom to be gained from homœopathic watchful waiting. It requires practitioners to thoroughly educate patients about this unusual aspect of the natural healing process before treatment starts. Intelligent, watchful waiting allows the patient's vital force to work unhindered. It prevents practitioners

---

[130] *Kent's new Remedies Clinical Cases Lesser Writings Aphorisms and Precepts,* compiled by Dr. W.W. Sherwood

from inadvertently interrupting and spoiling the curative response of the vital force to the well-chosen remedy, and avoids muddles. If we feel under pressure to act by impatience or fear rather than knowledge and reason, we lose the ability to think clearly and observe some small, yet extremely significant shift in symptoms that indicates exactly how the vital force is affected by the medicine.

Purposeful watchful waiting always demands careful consideration of both the context of the symptoms and whether or not they are life threatening. Patient safety is the priority. Commonsense must prevail. The patient's consent to watch and wait is always required. Where circumstances allow, if in doubt about what to do, pause and meticulously examine the patient and your casework. Knowledgeable waiting often avoids unnecessary patient suffering. Think carefully about why you are taking the action you have decided upon, and make sure you can explain it in such a way the patient understands exactly what is happening and why. Where appropriate, non-medicinal adjunctive measures may be offered to support patients during a waiting period.

Watchful waiting rules within the context of patient safety:

- Where possible, the reflex action of all practitioners should be to watch and wait with a purpose
- Waiting must be governed by knowledge. To know waiting is right is quite different from waiting without a fixed purpose. [131]
- There is no fixed time for waiting. Depending on the state of the individual's vital force and the nature of the disturbance experienced, it may be seconds, minutes, hours, days, weeks, months or even years
- The length of (waiting) time is not as important as being on the safe side, and waiting is the only safe thing to do. [132]

---

[131] Ibid

[132] Ibid

- Before making the next prescription, wait long enough for the original symptoms to return. That indicates the last dose is no longer affecting the vital force and it needs more help. It is calling for the same medicine in a slightly modified dose. Go to the next higher potency.
- If in doubt, wait for clarity. Re-examine the case to confirm or deny the accuracy of the previous prescription.

The next three chapters provide examples of Watchful Waiting plus in depth analysis of vital force responses to homœopathic medicines. Chapters 9 and 10 cover responses to centesimal potency responses only, and Chapter 11 covers LM/Q potency responses. Common confusion and mistakes will be identified and clarified, and useful case management guidelines offered.

9

Curative Response Analysis

The reader will note very carefully that the response analysis method applied in this book relates specifically to Hahnemann's homœopathic practice methodology and not any other divergent methodologies.

This chapter and Chapter 10 discuss responses to *centesimal potency doses only* because that potency scale is the one most frequently used.

In the treatment of longstanding illness, proper intervals between centesimal doses vary from 30 to 50 days or more. In first aid, urgent care treatment proper intervals are 5, 10, 20 or 30 minutes.

In response to centesimal potency doses of homœopathic medicines, Hahnemann states each patient's vital force has the potential to react in the following *favourable*, curative ways: [133]

- A rapid improvement of the patient *without* an intensification of symptoms
- A rapid short, and strong intensification of symptoms, then rapid improvement of the patient
- Original existing characteristic symptoms worsen, yet the patient feels better

---

[133] Dr. S. Hahnemann, *The Chronic Diseases: Their Peculiar Nature and Their Homœopathic Cure*

- Original characteristic symptoms come and go, yet the patient feels well overall
- Disappearance or amelioration of existing original characteristic symptoms followed by return of original symptoms
- Natural direction of cure
- Only original characteristic localised symptoms remain
- Original symptoms come and go, then come to a standstill
- Curative response followed by *possible* change in Original Characteristic Individualising Symptom Portrait

To avoid common errors such as jumping to wrong conclusions about what has happened and complicating a simple illness by re-prescribing too early or too frequently, selecting the wrong dose or incorrectly changing remedies, it is vital to curb over-enthusiasm, anxiety and the all-too-common, knee-jerk 'need to do something —anything' response. The task is to discover and accurately evaluate exactly what happened to the patient after each prescription and confidently make sense of all aspects of different vital force responses. In every aspect of homœopathic treatment, the patient's vital force is in control and it is that that the practitioner must listen for and observe. Decisions and actions during progress evaluation and analysis involve a thoughtful balancing act between waiting and prescribing: weighing the need for another dose against the need to wait and watch for further instructions from the vital force about the next action.

Let's explore typical vital force curative responses in detail.

Rapid improvement of the patient, *without* intensification of symptoms [134]

The patient returns and reports: 'I took the medicine and all my troubles disappeared. I feel like a million dollars. I didn't even have the twinge of anything you mentioned I might have.'

---

[134]Dr. J.T.Kent, *Lectures on Homœopathic Philosophy*

Evaluation:

This is an ideal response to a remedy and dose. The remedy affected the vital force and gave it exactly the right amount of assistance to finish the curative job it had started. This 'no aggravation with recovery of patient' response indicates the both the remedy and potency exactly fitted the case.

When disease affects the operation of the body rather than the structure, or in the beginning of acute diseases affecting the organs accompanied by severe pain, administration of the correct remedy and dose may be followed by rapid disappearance of symptoms without any aggravation. This is the most satisfactory kind of cure, pleasing alike to physician and patient. Remedy and potency were both exactly right.[135]

The initial response was imperceptible, yet the patient recovers steadily. According to doctors James. T. Kent and Herbert Roberts, conscientious followers of Hahnemann, 'No aggravation with recovery of the patient' responses may indicate that the chronic disease experienced belongs to the function of the nerves rather than threatened tissue changes. Although patients may suffer severely in these neurological illnesses before homœopathic treatment, they are often cured without experiencing the commonly observed initial short-lived intensification of symptoms. Providing the original symptoms do not return, the patient continues to feel better mentally, emotionally and physically, and their health is restored in an orderly way according to the correct direction of cure.

Action:

Celebrate! Improvement is in progress. Therefore, another remedy cannot be given. To administer another dose of remedy at this time would risk interrupting the curative response.

Wait watchfully for the reappearance of original symptoms to indicate the vital force is calling for further assistance to continue the curative response. Before making another prescription, let the

---

[135] Dr. S. Close, *The Genius of Homœopathy*

vital force continue its cycle of cure uninterrupted. While the patient experiences these trivial symptoms, wait until they report a definite return of old symptoms. Sometimes they may not return as severely as they did before the remedy was taken. The vital force 'whispers' rather than shrieks a request for more help. The practitioner must grow elephant ears so as not to miss the call.

Watchful waiting requires setting a series of progress reports at definite short intervals so that the correct time for the next dose may be known promptly. For example, at some point the patient's energy may take a dive without any reason, or the original symptoms might return somewhat changed from their former troublesome state. Either way, they trouble the patient again so you need to be aware of them.

Provided the patient does not experience any *new* symptoms, if original symptoms reappear, this is the time to consider repeating that exact same medicine—because it affected the vital force beneficially. To keep pace with the vital force's slightly increased energy and to continue to assist the vital force to the fullest extent possible, the medicine should be administered in a slightly modified ascending dose. For example, where the first dose is 30c, the next ascending dose is 200c.

Rapid short strong intensification of original symptoms, then rapid improvement of patient

The patient returns and reports: 'I took the remedy and everything got much worse on all levels for about a week or ten days. Then, during the last three weeks, the symptoms I originally complained about gradually disappeared. My spirits lifted, my mind is clearer, the pain in my neck has gone, there is still a bit of elbow pain, and there is a rash of some kind on my leg. Overall I feel okay and really, the rash doesn't bother me all that much.'

Evaluation:

Experience shows that when for several days there has been an improvement, half hours or whole hours or several hours will again appear when the case seems to become worse; but these period, so long as only the original ailments are renewed and no new, severe symptoms present themselves, only show a continuing improvement, being homœopathic aggravations which do not hinder but advance cure, as they are only renewed beneficent assaults on the disease, though they are wont to appear at times sixteen or twenty or twenty four days after taking a dose of antipsoric medicine.

These attacks, however, if the antipsoric remedy was selected fittingly and homœopathically and the dose was a moderate one, during its continued action take place ever more and more rarely and more feebly, but if the doses were too strong they come more frequently and more strongly, to the detriment of the patient.

This brief, moderate intensification of the original symptoms followed by rapid improvement and no new symptoms of any kind appear, indicates the medicine acts deeply into the very essence of the disease and that consequently it will be more effective in the future and that the illness is curable.[136]

Improvement will be marked, the reaction of the economy (the vital force) is vigorous and there is no tendency to any structural change in the vital organs. Any structural change that may be present will be found on the surface in organs that are not vital; abscesses will form and often glands that can be done without will suppurate in regions that are not important to the life of the patient. Such organic changes are surface changes, and are not like the changes that take place in the liver, in the kidneys, in the heart, and in the brain... A quick short strong aggravation is one that is wished for and is followed by quick improvement.[137]

After taking the remedy, the best case scenarios are a) where the administration of the remedy is followed by no aggravation whatever, or b) when the original symptoms of the illness are *briefly* intensified, excited, irritated, then gradually lessen, and the patient gradually improves overall. This so-called homœopathic

---

[136] Dr. S. Hahnemann, *The Chronic Diseases: Their Peculiar Nature and Their Homœopathic Cure*

[137] Dr. J.T. Kent, *Lectures on Homœopathic* Philosophy

aggravation is a sign that cure is beginning to happen, and that it may be expected with certainty.

Action:

Therefore, having been accurately chosen to suit the symptoms, that medicine should be allowed to continue and exhaust its action undisturbed without the least medicinal substance being given between doses.

However, in very tiresome ailments, these good results may not appear until the twenty-fourth or thirtieth day. In this situation, the dose will not have exhausted its favourable action until about the fortieth or fiftieth day. Therefore, it would be injudicious and an obstruction to the progress of the cure to consider giving any other medicine *before the fortieth or fiftieth day.* Once a symptom-similar medicine has been selected, given in the appropriate potency and proper dose *as a rule,* the physician should allow it to finish its action without disturbing it by giving an intervening remedy.

> It is a fundamental rule in the treatment of chronic diseases: To let the action of the remedy, selected in a mode homœopathically appropriate to the case of disease which has been carefully investigated as to its symptoms, come to an undisturbed conclusion, so long as it visibly advance cure and the while improvement still perceptibility progresses. This method forbids any new prescription, any interruption by another medicine and forbids as well the immediate repetition of the same remedy.

> ...A cure cannot be accomplished more quickly and surely than by allowing the suitable antipsoric to continue its actions so long as the improvement continues, even if this should be several, yea, many days beyond the assigned, supposed time of its duration, so as to delay as long as practicable the giving of a new medicine.

> Whoever can restrain impatience at this point, will reach the objective more surely and with more certainty.

> While a well-chosen medicine is acting and the patient someday feels a moderate headache, or perhaps a sore throat arises, or diarrhoea or else some moderate ailment or pain in one part or another, etc., these 'false' symptoms are an excitation of something which perhaps had been

more frequently troublesome before. They may continue for a few more days or they may return, but they will soon end.[138]

Therefore, do not consider making a second prescription.

The above favourable responses form the basis of Hahnemann's golden fundamental rule of homœopathic practice mentioned above related to proper intervals between doses: so long as the remedy and dose administered visibly advances cure, *even though a symptom changes slightly*, and improvement perceptibly progresses, let the action of the remedy come to an undisturbed conclusion. This method forbids any new prescription, any interruption by another medicine and forbids the immediate repetition of the same remedy.[139]

The patient's positive response indicates that they received the correct remedy and dose. So long as the curative response continues according to the inside-to-outside natural direction of cure, it should not be repeated. This rule applies even though the slightly changed symptoms would make it impossible for the first remedy to have been selected initially.

So long as improvement continues and symptoms that return are neither dangerous nor painful, hold fast to that first selected remedy. At correct intervals indicated by the reappearance of original symptoms, the same medicine may be repeated. Each subsequent dose can be slightly modified; ascending through the graduated scale of potencies, as the return of original symptoms indicates the power of each dose becomes exhausted. When the end of the potency scale is reached, if the vital force is still calling for the same remedy, commonsense indicates resume and re-ascend the scale from the point at which you started. For example, if the first dose was a 30c, resume the scale with a 30c; likewise, if you started with a 200c, resume with a 200c dose. The vital force, in its improved state, will respond curatively again.

---

[138] Dr. S. Hahnemann, *The Chronic Diseases: Their Peculiar Nature and Their Homœopathic Cure*

[139] Ibid

Original characteristic symptoms worsen, yet the patient feels better

After taking the remedy, the patient reports: 'My hot flashes are much worse, but I feel great!'

Evaluation:

There is significant improvement in the patient's general sense of well-being, in spite of the fact an original symptom intensified.

This response indicates that the remedy has affected the vital force and the patient is experiencing the so-called 'homœopathic aggravation', more accurately described by Hahnemann as the 'initial excitation response' of the vital force to the remedy, which usually occurs in acute illnesses and if the remedy dose has been too large.

> ...Usually, when the dose has not been sufficiently small and where the dose has been somewhat too large, immediately after ingestion—for the first hour, or a few hours—the remedy causes a slight aggravation that so much resembles the original disease, that it seems to the patient that it is an aggravation of the illness. In reality it is nothing more than an extremely similar medicinal disease, somewhat exceeding the original affection in strength.[140]

> In the treatment of acute diseases, the smaller the dose of homœopathic remedy, so much shorter is this apparent increase of the disease during the first hours.[141]

> But as the dose of a homœopathic remedy can scarcely ever be made so small that it shall not be able to relieve, overpower, indeed completely cure and annihilate the uncomplicated natural disease of not long standing that is analogous to it (§249, note), we can understand why a dose of an appropriate homœopathic medicine, not the very smallest possible, does always dose, during the first hour of its ingestion, produce a perceptible homœopathic aggravation of this.[142]

---

[140] Dr. S. Hahnemann, *The Organon of Medicine*, Sixth edition §157

[141] Ibid §159

[142] Ibid §160.

When I here limit the so-called homœopathic aggravation, or rather the primary action of the homœopathic medicine that seems to increase somewhat the symptoms of the original disease, to the first or few first hours, this is certainly true with respect to diseases of a more acute character and of recent origin; but where medicines of long action have to combat a malady of considerable or very long standing, where no such apparent increase of the original disease ought to appear during treatment and it does not so appear if the accurately chosen medicine was given in proper small, gradually higher doses, each somewhat modified with renewed dynamization (§247). [Which refers to 50-millesimal potency dosing method]. Such increase of the original symptoms of a chronic disease can only appear at the end of treatment when the cure is almost or quite finished.[143]

Action:

Wait watchfully. Leave the patient alone. Let the remedy continue to act and encourage the patient's vital force to vent the dynamic, inner disturbance out through the physical body. To avoid unnecessary suffering, compare the degree of symptom intensity and direction of cure of the symptoms with the intensity and location of the same symptoms at the time of presentation. As Hahnemann states: this initial intensification response is more likely to occur in urgent care, acute illnesses. It could be very brief, and should be followed by clear improvement of patient and symptoms.

If this response has occurred in a chronic illness, arrange for the patient to check in with you at least once a week to ensure this initial intensification response abates promptly.

If you are new to homœopathy and the waiting seems scary, establish regular, brief review consultations at more frequent intervals. This may be time-consuming, but nevertheless it builds confidence.

Symptoms that intensify in response to a dose of medicine that is too strong will subside in time. Errors in case management are unfortunate, but they offer valuable learning opportunities so long as they are rapidly identified, understood, corrected and recorded for further study. In this instance, the lesson learned is: selecting

---

[143] Ibid §161

the next potency for that patient, or the first potency for a different patient, demands deeper thought about which potency is most suitable and why. The best potency selections are made when the optimal minimal dose to effect cure fixed fundamental principle of homœopathy is applied (see Chapter 1, Proper Dose: Single Substance Single Dose).

Wait for the eventual return of the original symptoms indicating the effect of the remedy has ceased, before considering a further prescription is required.

When considering aggravations, it is essential to distinguish between the two types:

1. An aggravation of the disease, in which the patient and the pathological symptoms grow worse—a negative response requiring intervention

2. An aggravation of the characteristic, individualising symptoms of the patient, in which the intensified symptoms moved centrifugally, inward outwards, in the correct direction of cure: from more-vital to less-vital organs, and the patient improves. This is a curative response, not requiring intervention

Original characteristic symptoms come and go, yet the patient feels well overall

After taking the remedy the patient returns and reports one of the following:

'Everything I complained about went away for a while, and then they came back. The odd thing is, I feel well.'

A patient who has previously experienced genital herpes says, 'I feel well, except that the herpes I had before keeps coming back from time to time. Anyway, even that is better. It isn't quite as bad as it was before the medicine. Maybe the herpes lasts a day or an hour or less. My old attacks lasted weeks.'

Evaluation:

The original symptoms disappear and reappear from time to time. The remedy has affected the vital force, acted well and usefully, and penetrated deeply into the very essence of the disease. The tumultuous coming and going of characteristic symptoms indicates the vital force is restoring order and the curative response is continuing. We are witnessing a return of the original symptoms in a less frequent or less intense form compared to before the remedy was taken. In the example of the patient with genital herpes, each attack was less intense than previously. The symptom gradually grew weaker while the patient improved. These are homœopathic aggravations of the original ailments. They are assaults on the disease by the medicine. They do not hinder; they advance cure. If the dose is a moderate one, these excitations of the disease will take place ever more and more rarely and more feebly.[144] The reappearance of these moderately bothersome symptoms does not indicate repetition of the first prescription or that a different remedy for each of the symptoms is required.

Action:

Wait watchfully. Hahnemann explains why: Having chosen the homœopathic medicine most suited to the morbid symptoms, the physician should, as a rule, allow it to finish its action without disturbing it by administration of an intervening remedy. Before repeating the medicine, delay as long as practicable. So long as improvement continues, even if this should be several or many days, cure cannot be accomplished more quickly and surely than by allowing the suitable remedy to continue its action. Only when the original symptoms which had been eradicated or very much diminished, are renewed, begin to rise again for a few days, or again become perceptibly experienced, has the time surely come

---

[144] Dr. S. Hahnemann, *The Chronic Diseases: Their Peculiar Nature and Their Homœopathic Cure*

when another dose of the medicine should be given.[145] He gives this example:

> In a case where *sepia* had shown itself to be completely homœopathically antipsoric for a peculiar headache that appeared in repeated attacks, and where the ailment had been diminished both as to intensity and duration, while the pauses between the attacks had also been much lengthened, when the attacks re-appeared, I repeated the dose, which then caused the attacks to cease for one hundred days (consequently its action continued that long), when it reappeared to some degree, which necessitated another dose, after which no other attack took place for, now, seven years, while the health was also otherwise perfect.[146]

Hahnemann's Sepia case is a clear example of the curative power and wisdom of waiting. He continues his guidance:

> As a rule, therefore, the antipsoric medicine in chronic diseases continue their action the longer, the more tedious the diseases are... The physician must, therefore, in chronic diseases, allow all antipsoric remedies to act, thirty, forty or even fifty and more days *by themselves*, so long as they continue to improve the diseased state perceptibly to the acute observer, even though gradually; for so long the good effects continue with the indicated doses and these must not be disturbed and checked by any new remedy.

> In acute diseases, medicines act only a short time—the more acute the disease, the shorter the action.

> If appropriately selected medicines are not allowed to act their full time when they are acting well, the whole treatment will amount to nothing. If another remedy is administered too early, before the present remedy completes its action, or a new dose of the same remedy is given, the good effect of the preceding remedy will be lost and cannot be replaced because its complete action has been interrupted.[147]

---

[145] Ibid

[146] Dr. S. Hahnemann, *The Chronic Diseases: Their Peculiar Nature and Their Homœopathic Cure*

[147] Ibid.

The fundamental progress evaluation golden rule applies: so long as the remedy and dose administered visibly advances cure and improvement perceptibly progresses, allow the action of the remedy (which has been) selected carefully according to its symptom-similarity, come to an undisturbed conclusion. Giving another medicine immediately is forbidden.[148]

Disappearance or amelioration of existing original symptoms, followed by return of original symptoms

After the remedy is taken, the patient returns and reports: 'I was much better and now I am worse again.'

Evaluation:

This favourable response is a subtle variation of the previous response.

The first prescription was correct: the case is curable; the remedy assisted the vital force. The patient reports improvement, the symptoms disappeared, and then improvement ceases with the reappearance of the original symptoms. For this patient, the dose was insufficient to complete permanent restoration of health and the return of the original symptoms indicate the vital force is calling for further assistance.

Action:

Wait watchfully for a few days. Keep in touch with the patient. If the reappearing symptoms come and go intermittently with minimal disruption, then the vital force is still responding. Before repeating the prescription, the vital force must be observed to be truly exhausted, which is indicated by the persistence of the reappearing original symptoms. Only then may the previous remedy be repeated, and always in a slightly modified dose.

> Wait for the curative impulse to entirely subside and the reappearance, one by one, of original characteristic symptoms, falling into place

---

[148] Ibid

before the intelligent physician, to arrange an image of the disease for cure.

When the symptom picture, image returns unaltered, except for the absence of one or more symptoms, the first remedy should never be changed until ascending potencies have exhausted their powers.[149]

The rule is: *never change the remedy so long as the patient improves after administration of the medicine. If the patient feels improved, continue that remedy at appropriate intervals.* In this way we gradually increase the curative power of the vital force. That remedy should not be changed so long as the curative action can be maintained, until there are good reasons for changing it.

Many physicians say: 'If the symptoms change, I change the remedy.' That is one of the most detrimental things that can be done. Change the remedy if the symptoms have changed, providing the patient has not improved; but if the patient has improved, though the symptoms have changed, continued that remedy so long as the patient improves. Very often the patients are giving forth symptoms long forgotten. The patient has not heard them, or has not felt them because he has become accustomed to the, like the ticking or striking of the clock on the wall. Many of the symptoms that appear, and the slightest changes that occur, are old symptoms coming back. The patient is not always able to say that they are old symptoms retuning, but finally the daughter or somebody in the house will delight you by saying that her mother had these things years ago and she has forgotten them. So long as the curative can be obtained, and even though symptoms have changed, provided the patient is improving, hands off.[150]

As indicated by the patient's vital force, go up through the potencies of your chosen scale until you give a higher potency without effect. If you reach the end of the scale and the same remedy is still indicated, return to your starting potency and resume ascending the scale. The less encumbered vital force is more susceptible at a deeper level, to the ascending scale the second time around. Continuously improving with

[149] Kent's *New Remedies, Clinical Cases, Lesser Writings, Aphorisms and Precepts*, compiled by Dr. W.W. Sherwood

[150] Dr. J. T. Kent, *Lectures on Homœopathic Philosophy*

each modified dose, the remedy takes a stronger hold of the organism and the patient's health to a higher level of cure.[151]

Natural direction of cure

The patient returns and reports: 'My knee is more painful, I have pimples, but I'm sleeping better and I feel much less irritable than before.'

Evaluation:

Some symptoms are better; some are worse. The remedy affected the vital force and the symptoms are moving in the correct curative direction: innermost ('sleep has improved') to outermost ('pimples on skin') and head-to-toe ('knees are worse'). The disturbance at the centre is moving outwards and downwards. Cure is going in an orderly manner.

Action:

Wait watchfully. Carefully assess the shift in location and direction of all symptoms. Never risk interrupting the curative response by prescribing too early before the vital force signals it needs further help. If the repetition of a remedy is too early, the vital force is derailed or overwhelmed, and this prevents progress. While the symptom picture is in motion, leave the patient alone. While you are waiting, educate the patient about body's natural orderly way of healing itself.

The physician must wait for permanency or firmness in the relations of the image before making a prescription. Some say, 'I must give the patient medicine or he will go and see someone else.' I have only to say that it were better had all sick folks gone somewhere else, for these doctors seldom cure but often complicate the sickness.[152]

---

[151] Dr. S. Hahnemann, *Chronic Diseases: Their Peculiar Nature and Their Homœopathic Cure*

[152] Kent's *New Remedies, Clinical Cases, Lesser Writings, Aphorisms and Precepts*, compiled by Dr. W.W. Sherwood

Only original localised symptoms remain

The patient returns and reports: 'It's been a while now and overall I feel good. Bit by bit everything has improved, but I still have this patch of really irritating eczema on my tummy that won't go away, and the joint pains are there on and off.'

Evaluation:

The vital force has been left alone without interference; most of the original characteristic symptoms have been eliminated, but a few exterior localised symptoms remain affecting the limbs and skin. The disturbance at the centre has shifted from the interior to the exterior. The localised symptoms are in the physical sphere versus the mental sphere. The symptoms that are not bothering the patient very much are acting as a tolerable vent. Cure has been continuous but it is not quite finished. The vital force has responded well, but it might need either another dose, or new state might be emerging, indicating the need for a different remedy to complete the cure.

Action:

Wait actively for a week to ten days. Direct patient to report any changes if they occur in the interim. Then check for any changes. If there are no changes, and if the original symptoms persist, but are still tolerable, leave the vital force alone. When the symptoms intensify and trouble the patient again, the vital force is calling for further assistance. As there are no new symptoms, repetition of the first prescription is required in an ascending potency.

After a proper interval, if nothing has changed and the symptoms remain in their intensified state without improvement, another remedy is required. At this stage, we do not yet have any indication what that might be because the original symptom totality remains unchanged except for the improvement that has occurred up to a point, so until new symptoms appear, we must continue to wait. Explaining the reason for waiting to the patient will alleviate any impatience. Eventually something will change and the changes will guide us to the new remedy that suits both the original state with the new one.

Original symptoms come and go, then come to a standstill [153]

After the remedy was taken, there was an initial reaction in which the original symptoms intensified temporarily. Then, the turmoil gradually subsided until the patient has no symptoms and says, 'My symptoms have gone, I don't feel ill, but I don't feel well either, and I can't really say how I feel or why.'

Evaluation:

There is doubt about whether the vital force continues to respond to the remedy. The original symptoms appear to have lessened in their intensity and the patient has improved to some degree, but nothing seems to be happening now. The patient is most likely in the 'standstill phase' of recovery. If there are few or no clear symptoms, there is no clear guide to the next action.

Rarely is it the case that a new prescription becomes necessary when the case merely comes to a standstill. The first prescription has been made and the symptoms begin to change in an orderly way; they change and interchange and new symptoms come up, but finally the symptoms go back to their original state, not marked enough to be of any importance without any special suffering to the patient, and the patient has arrived at a state of standstill. The patient says: 'I have not symptoms, yet I am not improving; I seem to have come to a standstill position.' He says this about himself not about the symptoms.[154]

---

[153] Dr. J.T. Kent, *Lectures on Homœopathic Philosophy*

[154] Ibid

Action:

Wait watchfully. Examine the patient carefully; explore the potential of the symptoms having changed in an orderly way and receded to where the patient is not bothered by them. In this case, on closer inspection the chief complaint has improved, which is why the patient reports no symptoms. The patient and the symptoms have improved.

> It is the duty of the physician then to wait, and wait a long time... A new prescription cannot be entertained, because there is no guide to it ... Wait a long time when patients come to a standstill.

> The patient will get along just as well without any medicine, and get along better without the medicine that helped him than with it. In curable cases, whose prospects are good, he will go along for a long time, and become very much relieved of his symptoms.[155]

To avoid irrevocably spoiling excellent treatment, do not make another prescription. Allow the patient's vital force to rest without making another prescription.

Whenever in doubt, do not prescribe. Wait for a clear symptom image to emerge and the vital force to call for further assistance through uncomfortable changes experienced by the patient. At correct intervals, monitor the patient for a return of original symptoms. In acute conditions, the waiting time will be shorter than in chronic illness. Clarity always occurs after waiting actively; given time the blurred picture clears, knowledge of what is happening increases and correct decisions are easier to make.

Avoid allowing impatience to induce an error, or imposing an arbitrary schedule of progress on the patient. The unique nature of a person's vital force, susceptibility, inherent predispositions to illness and respones to medicines, reign supreme as action indicators. It is impossible to predict when and for how long an individual's vital force will respond. It is safer and wiser to resist the temptation to prescribe again merely because of some unsubstantiated theoretical formula such as 'a certain potency of a

---

[155] Ibid

certain remedy acts for a certain period, and if it has not acted within that certain time-frame, the remedy must be changed'.

> The finest curative action I ever observed has begun sixty days after the administration of the single dose.[156]

For some practitioners, a lack of confidence makes it is difficult to always trust in an intangible entity such as the individual's spirit-like vital force. For homœopathy to be effective, it is essential to acknowledge that in sickness and health, it is only the individual's vital force that is in control of the organism. Observing and listening to the patient's vital force through its expression of symptoms is a practitioner's only reliable guide. If a remedy is repeated or changed too soon—before the action of the first prescription is exhausted—we risk interrupting the cycle of cure that is under way. We also risk causing a dangerous intermingling of drug symptoms with the patient's symptoms with the tragic consequence that the original, once-clear symptom image is obscured and muddled to such an extent it cannot be undone. For clarity to prevail, remember Hahnemann's rule when using the centesimal potency: *the remedy must always be allowed to act to its fullest extent.*

For continuous recovery to occur, knowledge of the proper interval between each dose is critical. Whenever another prescription is under consideration, be sure the patient's report indicates that the window of susceptibility to that medicine is open and the patient's vital force is calling for more assistance.

> ...The interval between doses stands next in importance only to the selection of the right remedy.[157]

Careless, casual, ineffective monitoring of the case, being too quick on the draw, too eager to act and the perfect moment for the next prescription is easily missed. To ensure perfect timing it may

---

[156] *Kent's New Remedies, Clinical Cases, Lesser Writings, Aphorisms and Precepts*, compiled by Dr. W.W. Sherwood

[157] Dr. H. Farrington, *Homœopathy and Homœopathic Prescribing*

be necessary to check the patient's state every few days. Select a few key characteristic symptoms for review rather than the complete list: e.g. a mental general, physical general and chief physical particular symptom for easy comparison. Continue to wait while the patient's overall wellbeing remains steady or improves. During the 'standstill' wait until the original symptoms return and bother the patient again before prescribing.

In uncertain situations, where no significant new symptoms appear and the original symptoms have not altered in any marked degree, except that the intensity has lessened, there is no guide to another action or remedy. All we can do is wait for the return of the original symptoms.

Curative response, followed by *possible* change in Original Characteristic Symptom Portrait

After the first prescription, there has been an amelioration of symptoms and continued improvement for two or three ascending potency doses, which were given at the proper intervals. After the third or fourth dose of the remedy, the patient's vital force does not respond. There is no improvement and no change in the symptoms, except for the appearance of a symptom not mentioned or experienced earlier by the patient.

Evaluation:

Until the last dose, the remedy had affected the vital force curatively. Since the previous dose, there has been no improvement. The 'new' symptom may be a return of an old symptom that the patient forgot about because it disappeared a long time ago and had not recurred. The appearance of a 'new' symptom at this stage may also indicate that, perhaps at the time of the original history taking and original case analysis, this particular information was unavailable and consequently the first case analysis did not represent the complete symptom totality of the patient's suffering. The first prescription reflected only part of the symptom totality rather than the complete totality. Therefore, the remedy selected took the patient part way along the road to recovery, but it was unable to hold the case through a series of potencies and cause complete cure. Patients seldom remember everything that has contributed to their illness during the history-taking interview. As the vital force retraces its steps it brings unresolved conditions to the surface for resolution. Little by little, during cure, the symptom totality perceived at the beginning of treatment may expand. Patients often require a series of carefully selected medicines administered as indicated by the symptom totality, one remedy at a time over a period, to achieve complete recovery. For example, Silica takes up the burden of cure where Pulsatilla left off. Or the typical symptoms of Calcarea Carbonica merge into those of Lycopodium.

Action:

Wait actively, to see if the 'new' symptom subsides on its own. Check in the *Repertory of the Homœopathic Materia Medica* to confirm or deny the presence of the current remedy in the grouping of remedies for that symptom. Also check for the symptom in Hahnemann's *Materia Medica Pura* and *The Chronic Diseases: Their Peculiar Nature and Their Homœopathic Cure*. If it is confirmed, it is a medicinal symptom. Left alone without repetition of the remedy, the 'new' symptom will disappear in time. When the original symptoms reappear, repeat the remedy in the next ascending potency.

Where the remedy given is not in the homœopathic *Materia Medica* or the group of medicines corresponding to the 'new' symptom in the repertory, it is understood to be a truly a new, never-experienced-before symptom. Left alone, it too may disappear gradually. Be cautious. It is so easy to spoil excellent prescriptions. If that symptom persists, and only if it bothers the patient a lot, re-examine the case analysis for errors, if none, consider adding that 'new' symptom to the original portrait. Re-work the case and see if a different medicine runs through all the symptoms and more accurately reflects the changed needs of the patient's vital force.

After administration of the new, well-chosen medicine, the patient will say, 'This new remedy acted like the first one did in the beginning.' Patients feel the medicine when it is acting, working properly.[158]

The above examples clearly illustrate how easy it is to overlook subtle differences and commit avoidable errors, including Hahnemann's three chief errors:[159]

- To consider a dose of homœopathic medicine to be too small.
- To choose an unsuitable homœopathic remedy.
- To not allow each dose of remedy to act its full time.

Commenting on these three chief errors Hahnemann says:

A dose can hardly be given too small, if the remedy was correctly selected according to the carefully investigated symptoms of the disease, and if everything in the diet and the remaining mode of life of the patient which would obstruct or counteract the action of the medicine is avoided, and if the patient does not disturb the remedy effects by violation of the rules. If ever it should happen that the choice of remedy has not been correctly made, the great advantage remains that the smallest dose of the incorrectly selected remedy will be counteracted more easily.

'As to the *second* chief error in the cure of chronic disease (*the unhomœopathic choice of the medicine*) the homœopathic beginner (many, I am sorry to say, remain beginners their whole life long) sins chiefly through inexactness, lack of earnestness and through love of ease.'

The *third* leading mistake which the homœopathic physician cannot too carefully not too steadfastly avoid while treating chronic disease, is in hastily and thoughtlessly—when a properly moderate dose of a well selected antipsoric medicine has been serviceable for several days—giving some other medicine in the mistaken supposition that so small a dose could not possibly operate and be of use more than eight or ten days.[160]

---

[158] *Kent's New Remedies, Clinical Cases, Lesser Writings, Aphorisms, and Precepts,* compiled by Dr. W. W. Sherwood.

[159] Dr. S. Hahnemann: *The Chronic Diseases: Their Peculiar Nature and Their Homœopathic Cure*

[160]Ibid

Experience indicates other avoidable practitioner mistakes are:

- Forgetting to educate patients concerning the patient-centred, patient-lead nature of homœopathy, which means that practitioners are extremely dependent on the patient's commitment to collaborate in the endeavour of health restoration.
- Forgetting to educate patients that the restoration of their health depends on their agreement to comply with various reasonable lifestyle changes.
- Forgetting to educate patients concerning the requirement for veracity when reporting back.

For the sake of clarity and to reduce unintentional extra patient suffering, before making a final decision or taking any action always:

- Keep calm
- Avoid haste
- Curb the love of ease
- Think before you act
- Ask yourself: exactly why am I doing what I am doing?'
- Consider carefully which fundamental principle(s) of homœopathic practice should be applied, given a particular set of response circumstances and required actions
- To provide irrefutable evidence for a specific action, use the patient's original verbatim descriptions of symptoms

Having identified and understood favourable, curative responses it's time to grapple with the vital force's far more challenging non-curative responses to centesimal potency doses.

10

Non-Curative Response Analysis

This chapter covers non-curative vital force responses to *centesimal potency doses only*. Typically, they fall into the following main categories:
- Non-curative direction of some original symptoms, improvement of others, and appearance of a possible new symptom.
- Overreaction
- No change in original symptoms
- Too short relief of symptoms
- Prolonged intensification of original symptoms followed by gradual improvement
- Prolonged intensification of original symptoms followed by patient worsening overall
- Original symptoms intensify followed by short interval of improvement then relapse
- Severe intensification of original symptoms, plus development of organic pathology
- Appearance of new symptoms

The following section discusses these categories with guidance on how to steady the faltering vital force.

Non-curative direction of *some* original symptoms improvement of others, and appearance of a possible new symptom

'My swollen inflamed knees and occasional hot flashes, which didn't used to bother me much anyway, have worsened; however, some of my irritating skin patches are better. At least the anxiety hasn't gotten worse because my concentration is down the tubes. I am more depressed than I was before the remedy, plus I feel my energy has drained away and my heart is going a mile a minute—I never had that before.'

Evaluation:

Some of the original symptoms affecting the physical region—which caused minor discomfort before the remedy—have become more uncomfortable after the remedy while other physical symptoms have improved. A possible 'new' symptom related to the heart has appeared. Emotional symptoms are unchanged or worse; intellectual function has deteriorated along with the physical energy.

This response indicates that overall in general the patient's vital force is weaker and moving in the non-curative direction. The disease is growing stronger; it is progressing inward and upward, from extremities to heart and brain, from less vital to more vital organs.

There are several reasons for this non-curative response:

• The first remedy selected fit only part of the patient's symptom totality rather than the complete totality; therefore, the remedy selection was incorrect. This circumstance is likely to be due to the central disturbance remaining undetected by the practitioner because the illness history was improperly taken, with the result that the symptom totality of the illness could not be perceived

- Prior medical mismanagement severely weakened the vital force and rendered it insufficient for recovery using homœopathy
- A well-chosen remedy was repeated too soon before the first dose had been exhausted, and the second dose interrupted the curative response to the first dose. Too frequent a repetition of a symptom-similar remedy often results in homœopathic symptom suppression
- A combination of all or any of these possibilities

Action:

In these alarming circumstances, resist panic. Pause, take a deep breath and calm yourself. THINK logically. Act methodically and urgently.

The non-curative response *must* be interrupted. Immediately restudy the situation and reanalyse the whole state of suffering again from its original beginnings through to the moment the patient presented for treatment. Detect and correct errors. Select a new remedy: one that has been proven to possess the power to induce similar symptoms that resemble the illness more closely. Consult the *Materia Medica* (homœopathic medicine experiment knowledge-base) again to confirm the accuracy of the remedy selection. Consider the current weakened state of the vital force and carefully choose a more suitable dose and proper intervals between doses. Explain to the patient how you arrived at the new remedy and why, and advise the patient regarding the dosing method. Set the next progress report date. Watch and wait. Stay alert. In treatment of longstanding illness, after taking the newly selected remedy, some patients return saying:

'I must be allergic or something to that last medicine; my skin is all inflamed.'

Don't risk being misled. Re-examine the patient closely regarding the original symptom totality. In the example given above, occasional flashes of heat and inflamed swollen knees experienced before the remedy had been replaced with frequent severe heart palpitations and depression, etc. If the new remedy and dose were correctly homœopathically selected, the burdensome symptoms associated with vital organs will disappear and be replaced by symptoms associated with a less vital organ, in this instance the skin. The more suitable homœopathic remedy induced a curative response; symptoms are beginning to move in the correct direction of cure—from the centre to the circumference. The vital force is back on track. Phew! Educate the patient concerning the correct direction of cure.

If the new remedy and dose does not produce a curative response, it must be concluded that the practitioner has not detected the central disturbance. The illness history was not taken properly. That particular practitioner confusion leaves the patient up the creek without a paddle. To aimlessly administer remedy after different remedy will not bring about cure. It is a mistake that is likely to induce a terrible muddle and could render the patient close to being beyond cure.

> Too often the remedy has been only similar enough to the superficial symptoms to change the totality and the image comes back altered, therefore resembling another remedy, which must always be regarded as a misfortune, by which the case is sometimes spoiled, and the hand of the master may fail to correct the wrong done.[161]

Such an unfavourable response highlights the need to avoid the common error of prescribing remedies for single or few symptoms, prescribing for only part of the symptom totality, or perhaps prescribing many different unsuitable medicines for each of the changing symptoms. After prescribing more than one remedy without achieving a curative response, especially in acute conditions, stop. Applying this rule is much more difficult that just doing something and giving a badly chosen remedy that does not correspond to the essential symptoms of the case because you do not know the patient's essential symptoms. Learn how to wait and observe, and don't lose your head.

---

[161] *Kent's New Remedies, Clinical Cases, Lesser Writings, Aphorisms, and Precepts,* compiled by Dr. W. W. Sherwood

In order to avoid further patient suffering and get the patient back on the path to recovery, it is wiser for practitioners to swallow their pride and seek patient consent to discuss the case with a more experienced colleague. In that way, patient and practitioner anxiety is decreased, faulty case management procedures are rapidly identified and corrected, and the patient is given a greater opportunity to recover.

When patients experience the **Non-curative direction** response, it is only a practitioner's clarity of thought, intelligence, understanding and rigorous application of the fixed fundamental principles of homœopathy, meticulously maintained records, and proper case analysis methodology, that saves the day.

Overreaction

Four or five weeks after taking the remedy, the patient returns and reports that some or all of the original symptoms are worse.

Evaluation

This is a very complicated situation. Haste is the enemy here. There are five possible evaluations for this response:
- wrong medicine was selected;
- dose was very close to a physiological dose and too violent
- extreme susceptibility, hypersensitivity to selected remedy;
- dose too high or too strong.

Bring your mind to order. Take your time to think carefully about which of those options options applies your particular patient's situation.

Evaluation 1: Wrong remedy

The remedy selected is completely incorrect, or suited to only a portion of the symptom totality.

Action:

Restudy the case to find a more appropriate remedy. Be careful about selecting the dose. Hahnemann reassures us:

If it should ever happen that the choice of remedy has been incorrectly made, it may be more easily counteracted with a more suitable medicine, if the remedy is always given in the smallest dose to effect cure. [162]

Evaluation 2: Dose too close to a physiological dose.

The correct symptom-similar remedy was given in a too crude dose. This means that dose contains physiological molecular material of the medicinal substance remains in the dose. For example, when using the centesimal potency scale, the low 6c, 9c, and 12c potencies were administered. Hahnemann says perhaps it was also administered frequently and repeatedly. The action of the too large dose of medicine will be decided, determined, in the first sixteen, eighteen or twenty days after being taken.[163]

According to Hahnemann, on subsequent days, if the same irritated original symptoms appear at the same strength as at the beginning or even with increased severity, it is a sign that although the remedy was correctly selected according to homœopathic principles, the dose of that remedy was too large, and it is understood that no cure will be effected by that remedy. The medicine was given in such a large dose it has established a disease, which in some respects is similar to the original one. However, in its present intensity, that medicine also unfolds (releases, produces) its other symptoms, which invalidates the symptom-similarity. Instead of producing the former symptom-similar chronic disease, without extinguishing the former old original one it produces a dissimilar indeed a more severe and troublesome one.

---

[162] Dr. S. Hahnemann: *The Chronic Diseases: Their Peculiar Nature and Their Homœopathic Cure*

[163] Ibid

Action:

Hahnemann's advice is as follows: The injurious medicinal drug disease will need to be extinguished by stopping the action of the medicine. This is accomplished either by selecting and administering a known antidote, or, if this is not known, giving another medicine that fits the patient's state more closely. This time give it in a *very moderate dose*. If this action does not extinguish the medicinal disease and neither patient nor symptoms improve, restudy the case and search for another remedy as homœopathically suitable as possible.

> I have experienced this accident, which is very obstructive to cure and cannot be avoided too carefully. Still ignorant of the strength of its medicinal power, I gave Sepia in the too large a dose. This trouble was still more manifest when I gave Lycopodium and Silica in the billionth degree four to six poppy seed pellets.

> When the stormy assault caused by too large (meaning too crude) dose of a homœopathically selected medicine has been assuaged through administration of another, better-selected remedy, the same remedy that had been hurtful only because of its overlarge dose, can be used again in the case with the greatest success, when it is homœopathically indicated; *but this time, only if it is given in a far smaller dose, in a much more highly potentized, attentuated, milder quality.*[164]

Thus Hahnemann tells us to administer a more refined, smaller highly diluted and agitated dose. For example, in the above case, consider a more highly refined, less disruptive, moderate potency such as 30c.

Evaluation 3: Extreme susceptibility

The individual is extremely susceptible or hypersensitive to the correctly selected remedy.

Action:

Assess the severity of the patient's oversensitivity to a well-chosen remedy. If the overreaction, oversensitivity is experienced

---

[164]Dr. S. Hahnemann: *The Chronic Diseases: Their Peculiar Nature and Their Homœopathic Cure*

as pain that rapidly drains away energy and weakens the vital force, examine the patient carefully to determine pain-tolerance levels. Assess the degree to which the pain troubles the patient. If the patient is reasonably comfortable enough to continue without resorting to adjunctive measures, let the vital force continue to work without interruption. So long as the remedy is not repeated, the pain will gradually disappear. To confirm the pain is decreasing, monitor the patient closely.

If the pain, or any other symptom that arose after taking the remedy, has never occurred with this intensity before and it is extremely burdensome, Hahnemann advises that, in such a case those symptoms are a sign that the medicine was not selected in the correct homœopathic manner and they are not to be endured. The response of the vital force, the action of the remedy must be stopped by either: (a) giving an antidote if it is known, or (b) in its place, giving another medicine more accurately related to the symptoms of the chronic illness.[165]

If you elect to replace the remedy, it is necessary to obtain as much information about the exact nature of burdensome symptoms as possible. It is especially important to elicit all the individualising, modifying features of that symptom. In the desire to correct one error, be very careful to avoid committing another very common error: don't focus on the intensified state alone and select a remedy based on a single symptom or too few symptoms in isolation of the symptom totality. Commission of that mistake risks the vital force removing that intensified symptom without resolving it. Unresolved, it may disappear for a while; however, it will reappear, adding a different muddle to the current one. Whenever a case is restudied it is wise to always view the case from the perspective of symptom *totality*. Using the expanded information, consult the Repertory again carefully according to the new case analysis. Consult the *Materia Medica* to confirm that the symptom-similar remedy that appears at the end of the reanalysis definitely resembles the illness more closely than the previous

---

[165] Ibid

remedy selected, and that it reflects the whole state of the individual's suffering rather than merely a portion of it.

If the symptoms of this different remedy do not resemble the illness more closely, rather than make another imperfect remedy selection, talk to the patient about the difficulty you are experiencing. Explain that you need more information to guide you to the correct remedy. Ask the patient to persevere. Monitor them closely at four- to five-day intervals. Waiting actively often increases the likelihood for new information to emerge and be reported, which improves the opportunity for a more suitable remedy to be selected.

Simple illnesses are likely to resolve with the assistance of a single remedy and dose. Complex cases sometimes require a series of remedies and doses at proper intervals—each one capable of either taking the patient a little further along the road to complete recovery or countering vital force overreactions without interrupting curative responses. The properly conducted illness history consultation indicates illness simplicity or complexity.

Where it is necessary to change from one remedy to another, the vital force responds more favourably to those that are related to, or complement, the action of each other. The best source of this information is in Hahnemann's preamble to each medicine recorded in both his *Materia Medica Pura* and *The Chronic Diseases: Their Peculiar Nature and Their Homœopathic Cure.* A similar authoritative resource is Kent's *Lectures on Homœopathic Materia Medica.* For example, Hepar sulphuricum, Nux Vomica, Nitric Acid, Pulsatilla, Coffea, Chamomilla[166] and Camphora[167] are mentioned as remedies worthy of consideration when managing vital force overreactions. However, they should only be administered where the symptom totality fits the symptoms produced by the medicine. These medicines should never be administered routinely to calm over-reactions.

---

[166]Dr. J.T. Kent, *Lectures on Homœopathic Materia Medica*

[167] Dr. S. Hahnemann, *Materia Medica Pura,*

Practitioners of pure method homœopathy understand that illness is unique to each person, and that nothing about homœopathy is routine. It is a serious error of judgement to consider that a course of homœopathic remedies used for one individual and condition will restore health in all individuals with similar symptoms or conditions. Recommendations in professional homœopathic journals that certain illnesses demand a particular series of remedies be administered routinely in a particular sequence, dose and interval between doses is an excellent example of encouraging practitioners to slide backwards to the pernicious routinism of the old school that is as much the antithesis of homœopathy as night is to day.[168]

In homœopathy, the golden rule is: *never prescribe homœopathic medicines routinely or without careful forethought, and only if they suit the totality of the state of illness under consideration.*

Painful overreactions can be very distressing to experience and witness. Pain drains the strength of the vital force faster than anything. In both the short- and long-term, it can be very detrimental to the patient. There is often considerable pressure to do something to ease the suffering. Educate the patient thoroughly about what has happened and why. Instruct them to keep in touch. Immediately reanalyse the case and develop a more appropriate plan of homœopathic treatment. If you are struggling or confused, consider asking a more experienced practitioner for urgent help.

Evaluation 4: Hypersensitivity to selected remedy

The potency selected was too high for the weakened state of the vital force. High centesimal potencies, for example 1M upwards, penetrate deeply into the body and mind, which is why for gentlest cure to avoid the possibility of overreactions, it is wise to start lower down the centesimal potency scale and work up rather than start treatment with the very high potencies. According to Hahnemann:

---

[168] Dr. S. Hahnemann, *Organon of Medicine,* Sixth edition, Author's Preface

The signs of improvement in the disposition and mind, however, may be expected only soon after the medicine has been taken when the dose has been *sufficiently minute* (i.e., as small as possible), an unnecessarily larger dose of even the most suitable homœopathic medicine acts too violently, and at first produces too great and too lasting a disturbance of the mind and disposition to allow us to perceive an improvement in them.[169]

Action:

Don't panic! Stay calm. First: *think carefully*. Second: *act confidently*. At all costs we need to keep our heads in the midst of patient turmoil. Remember, whenever the vital force overreacts, the more cautiously we must go on. This is particularly applicable when the turmoil is great, the tissue change is deep, the reaction is intense or painful or the trouble is deep-seated.

The greatest sufferings may intervene in the change of symptoms during progress of permanent recovery, and if symptoms are disturbed by a new prescription or palliated by an inappropriate medicine, the patient may never be cured. [170]

Follow the action directions for managing non-curative responses to:

- Prolonged intensification of original symptoms followed by gradual improvement
- Prolonged original symptom intensification followed by worsening of the patient overall

Evaluation 5 Dose Too High:

This was covered in Evaluation 4 when we discussed the hypersensitivity of patients.

No change in original symptoms

Several weeks after taking the remedy, the patient returns and reports: 'Nothing has changed, I am exactly the same.'

---

[169] Dr. S. Hahnemann: *Organon of Medicine*, Sixth edition, §253 F/n 138

[170] *Kent's New Remedies, Clinical Cases, Lesser Writings, Aphorisms and Precepts*, compiled by Dr. W.W. Sherwood

Evaluation:

The first prescription was incorrect. If the correct medicine has been chosen but the potency was incorrect, there would have been a slight shift towards improvement albeit short lived.

Action:

Examine the patient thoroughly to verify the evaluation. Review all aspects of the original symptom totality to confirm beyond all doubt that the patient has experienced no change whatsoever in either the degree of energy or their original mental, emotional and physical disposition discomfort. Confirm each region of the body affected *before* the remedy remains as affected after the remedy and ensure no new symptoms have occurred.

If the information gathered verifies without a doubt that no changes have occurred, the conclusion is the remedy and dose selected was incorrect.

Educate the patient regarding what happened. Apologise for the error. Inform the patient that to rectify the error, the case requires further urgent study, which will start immediately.

Error correction is easiest and quickest if speculation is avoided. For comparison, orally provide the patient with the original basis for the first prescription: the symptom totality portrait and characteristic symptom hierarchy that formed the basis of the remedy selection. Refer to the patient's statements documented verbatim in the illness-history record. To clarify which part of the original illness portrait is incorrect, review the information using the patient's own symptom description language rather than the technical repertory rubric jargon of the case analysis.

Reviewing the original illness portrait with patients allows them to easily correct practitioner errors, and even shine new light on important aspects of their original illness that perhaps they previously considered to be insignificant.

If any new, never-before-experienced symptoms are unearthed, these may be symptoms that the medicine that had been prescribed had the power to induce, rather than signs that the illness is progressing. Use the *Materia Medica* to search for the new symptoms. If they are recorded in the *Materia Medica*, it is safe to conclude that they are medicinal symptoms and, if left alone, they will disappear on their own. Monitor the patient closely to confirm their disappearance.

Make sure to *exclude* any new symptoms in the reanalysis that occurred after the first remedy was taken. If this isn't done, any medicinal symptoms might be intermingled with characteristic symptoms of the original illness and another incorrect remedy will be selected. Having discovered all the errors, restudy the case meticulously from the beginning.

Should the reanalysis indicate that the remedy already administered remains the most symptom-similar to the illness, a different remedy cannot be given due to the fact that this is not indicated as the correct one.

In this perplexing situation, educate the patient as to the outcome of the reanalysis. Inform the patient that it is necessary to allow the vital force to call again for the first remedy. Watch and wait for it to produce a return of the original symptoms. This reappearance indicates that a repetition of the remedy that induced the unfavourable response is required again in a slightly modified dose.

How long should we wait?

There can be no routine period of waiting. It depends on the nature of the patient's vital force and the pace of the illness. Schedule progress reports at five-day intervals, and direct the patient to report any return of symptoms that may occur before a scheduled appointment.

Once the reappearance of the original symptoms occurs, the patient is given the next higher centesimal potency, or better still consider switching to the LM/Q potency scale.

Too short relief from symptoms

In treatment of a chronic illness, after ingesting the remedy the patient returns and reports: 'For a week or so some of the symptoms I had experienced before the remedy began to disappear and I felt better. Now those symptoms have stopped disappearing. What's going on?'

Evaluation:

> When the dose of a well-selected remedy that is in every way suitable and beneficial has made some beginning progress towards improvement, but then *after seven, ten or fourteen days or even fewer, the peculiar symptoms of the disease being treated visibly cease to diminish, that response indicates the improvement has manifestly come to a stop.*[171]

Action:

Reexamine the patient to confirm without doubt that there is no disturbance of the mind, and no appearance of any *new* troublesome symptoms. Where that situation is confirmed, it is prudent to wait for the vital force to signal clearly that it needs more help.

> In the treatment of chronic disease with a remedy selected carefully according to its symptom similarity, it is a fundamental rule: *To let the action of the remedy, carefully selected according to its symptom-similarity, come to an undisturbed conclusion, so long as it visibly advances cure and improvement perceptibly progresses.*
>
> This method forbids any new prescription, any interruption by another medicine and forbids the immediate repetition of the same remedy.[172]

To wait reduces the risk of accidentally overwhelming the vital force, interrupting the curative and spoiling the case by administering another dose of the remedy at the wrong time. To ensure the next dose is given at the proper time, schedule shorter interval progress reports.

Where reexamination of the patient reveals improvement has ceased *and* the original symptoms have reappeared, give an immediate repetition of the same medicine in a similarly small

---

[171] Dr. S. Hahnemann, *The Chronic Diseases: Their Peculiar Nature and Their Homœopathic Cure*

[172] Ibid

amount, but most safely in a different [higher] degree of dynamic potency.[173] The same remedy is indicated because its sphere of operation closely resembles the original symptom totality, which *has not changed.* The first potency selected was incorrect because it proved to be insufficient for complete recovery.

Remember:

> The practice of giving patients several doses of the same medicine to take with them, so that the patient may take them at certain intervals, without first considering whether this repetition may affect them injuriously or not, is negligent empiricism and unworthy of a homœopathic physician.

> In every case, a patient should not be allowed to take or be given a new dose of a medicine, without each patient's response being carefully reexamined and by so doing, the practitioner becomes convinced concerning whether it is useful or not to give a new dose.

For this very important reason:

> Suppose the patient experiences symptoms that are different and have never occurred before, or never in the way they are now, or they are trifling, or are peculiar to the medicine selected and not to be expected in the disease process. These symptoms frequently pass off without interrupting the helpful activity of the remedy, and the action of the remedy ought not to be interrupted.[174]

The reason that patient experienced those new or trifling symptoms is due to that particular patient's high degree of susceptibility to that particular remedy. To confirm that these 'not experienced before, or trifling symptoms' are part of the influence of the medicine on the vital force rather than signs of illness progression, consult the repertory. Search for each such 'trifling' symptom experienced. If the remedy administered appears in the group of remedies corresponding to each of those symptoms, its appearance in each grouping confirms that remedy has the power to induce that particular symptom or symptoms according to the homœopathic drug trial data concerning that particular medicine.

---

[173] Ibid

[174] Ibid

These 'new' symptoms are peculiar to that medicine. The patient's vital force should be left alone to continue its curative response. Without interruption of another dose of medicine, the 'trifling' symptoms will gradually disappear.

Sometimes patients might report a slight variation of the 'Too short relief of symptoms' response. Which looks like this:

> After a taking a high CM centesimal dose of deep acting remedy for a long standing illness, the patient returns and reports that at the end of the first, second and third weeks he did well and has been improving all the time from the remedy. At the end of the fourth week the patient returns and reports: 'I've been running down.'[175]

Evaluation:

This is an unfavourable response. Be suspicious. In a curable case where prospects are good, *provided a medicine was accurately selected,* after ingesting a very high centesimal dose, patients are relieved of their symptoms for a long time without needing another medicinal dose.

The most probable reasons for this particular unfavourable response are:

- Something occurred to interrupt the curative response.
- The first remedy selected was only partially symptom-similar rather than being totally symptom-similar and the dose was incorrect.
- There are significant structural changes going on; organs have been or are being destroyed, and they are in a very precarious condition.
- The curability of the patient was unclear or misperceived by the practitioner at the outset of treatment.

> In acute cases we may see this too short amelioration of the symptoms; for instance, a dose of medicine given in a violent inflammation of the brain may remove all the symptoms for an hour, and the remedy have to be repeated...and we find an amelioration of only thirty minutes. You may then make up your mind, that this patient is in a desperate condition, because it is too short an amelioration. In

---

[175] Dr. J. T. Kent, *Lectures on Homœopathic Philosophy*

acute states, if there is an amelioration of too short duration it is because such high grade inflammatory action is present, the organs are threatened by the rapid processes going on. [176]

Action:

Examine the patient to discover which of the possibilities apply. If patient examination reveals the curative response was interrupted—whether intentionally or unintentionally—by something (e.g. excessive intake of alcohol or drugs; excessive water, air or food deprivation; shock or trauma or excessive exposure to toxic substances or stress) consider whether the patient's life is under immediate threat. If the situation is not life threatening, *wait* for the effect of the interruptive influence to subside and for the patient's original symptoms to re-emerge. When that happens, it is safe to conclude the vital force is calling for more of the same medicine again, only this time in a slightly modified dose.

If patient examination reveals nothing has interfered with the curative response, it is safe to conclude the first remedy and dose was imperfectly selected because it suited only *part of* the illness rather than the symptom totality. The patient is moving in the non-curative direction (e.g. from outwards inward or from less vital organ to more vital organ). The illness is progressing; curability of the patient was doubtful at the outset but misperceived by the practitioner. The response must be interrupted.

Reanalyse the case immediately, making sure any new information concerning the original illness gleaned during the re-examination of the patient is included. Select a remedy that better reflects the symptom-similarity totality and select a dose that better suits the state of the patient's weakened vital force. Administer the new remedy and dose, and monitor the patient very closely, keeping alert for changes that indicate the patient is improving or worsening. Where these difficulties arise in emergency, acute illnesses, monitoring patients at short intervals of five to fifteen

---

[176] Ibid

minutes is required. Chronic illnesses will require at least weekly monitoring intervals.

For further information, review guidelines above concerning *Non-curative direction*

The following examples of vital force non-curative responses show the progressively complex nature of practitioner decision making processes which are required to help patients overcome setbacks and where possible, help a stumbling vital force get back on the path to recovery.

Prolonged intensification of original symptoms followed by gradual improvement[177]

After ingesting a very high (10M or higher) centesimal dose of a well-indicated remedy, a chronically ill patient returns and reports: 'The symptoms I was experiencing most recently before the remedy got worse for several weeks afterwards, then a slow and steady improvement on all levels occurred. Overall I feel moderately better.'

Evaluation:

Before the remedy was taken, the chronic state had the beginnings of marked tissue changes, but destructive changes in the vital organs had not yet occurred. The vital force's vain attempts to restore health unassisted left it severely weakened. This particular patient was on the borderline of curability, but the practitioner failed to recognise the signs. The prolonged original symptom intensification without the appearance of any new symptoms indicates that the practitioner misjudged the dose needed for the state of the vital force and improperly selected one that was too strong for such a severely weakened vital force. The

---

[177] Dr. J. T. Kent *Lectures on Homœopathic Philosophy*

improperly selected dose almost entirely overwhelmed the patient's vital force.

Action:

Inform the patient that a prescription error occurred and apologise. Explain that, to correct the mistake, it is necessary to WAIT actively to allow the vital force to continue the slow, steady improvement it has begun.

Monitor the patient closely for a week to ten days to confirm sufficiency of the vital force and that the steady improvement continues. If the evaluation and action are correct, the totality of symptoms will gradually subside or disappear according to the natural direction of cure.

Wait for the original symptoms to reappear and persist where possible for three or four days. Then, repeat the remedy at a dose that is extremely well thought through. Use one that is more similar in strength to the weakened vital force, and less likely to overwhelm it.

After that particular dose is ingested, monitor the patient closely. If the patient gradually feels a little better than before the first dose was taken, there is potential for the interior symptoms to have an outward manifestation and the patient go on to recover.

However, be warned: because the first dose was incorrect, sometimes the next dose causes the patient to experience a repetition of the previous adverse response. This often happens where the vital force is so seriously overwhelmed by the first improperly selected dose that the patient is now walking the tightrope of borderline curability. If the patient's health nose dives after taking the remedy again, it may be necessary to interrupt this second unfavourable response. This interruption is best managed by using a known antidotal remedy listed in the *Materia Medica*. If this action is necessary, exert great caution. Commission of another mistake could be disastrous. Think very carefully about which characteristic symptoms you select to represent the adverse response totality of symptoms; use only those symptoms that the patient describes clearly and about which you feel most confident.

Selection of the remedy should only be made where the symptom-similarity totality agrees, i.e. if the characteristic disagreeable symptoms experienced are similar to the characteristic symptoms artificially induced in healthy people by an antidotal remedy. Administer that remedy in the proper dose best suited to the vital force's weakened state.

It is a risky business to counter the effects of mistakes by switching medicines midstream. A complicated illness is very easily rendered more complicated. This is why:

> It is always well in doubtful cases to go to the lower potencies (30c – 200c), and in this way cautiously be prepared to interrupt the action of a medicine if the case takes the wrong direction. [178]

Prolonged intensification of original symptoms followed by patient worsening overall

A patient walks into the clinic, somewhat stoop-shouldered, with a hacking cough that he has had for a good many years...His face is sickly, he is lean, anxious, careworn; he is suffering from poverty, poor clothing and scanty food. You examine all his symptoms, which clearly indicate the need for an antipsoric remedy. From the case history you know he has needed the remedy for a good while...You examine his chest and discover that he does not have the expansion he ought to have, and you detect the presence of tuberculosis by feeble pulse and many other corroborating symptoms, and you ascertain that the patient has been steadily declining.

You give the medicine, after a few days he returns with quite a sharp aggravation of the symptoms; his cough has increased, he has night sweats and he is more feeble. Homœopathic physicians like to hear of an exacerbation of the symptoms; but this patient returns in a week and the aggravation is still present and somewhat on the increase. The patient's cough is worse, the expectoration is more troublesome than ever, his night sweats have continued. He returns at the end of the second week and he is still worse, and since he took that medicine all the symptoms have been worse. Before he took that medicine he was comparatively comfortable, but at the end of the fourth week he is steadily growing worse. There has been no amelioration following the

---

[178] Dr. J.T. Kent, *Lectures on Homœopathic Philosophy*

(initial) aggravation; he is evidently declining; now he is so weak he cannot come to the office.

- What have we done?[179]

Evaluation:

A mistake has been made. After taking the remedy, the patient experienced intensification of the original symptoms, without increased vitality or sense of well-being. The symptom excitation fails to subside and the patient's vitality and mental, emotional and physical condition progressively declines.

In the example given, when organic disease is present, there are many signs in the chest to make an intelligent physician doubt whether to give a deep remedy. In this instance, it is probable that the remedy has been administered too late. Due to insufficient prevailing vital force, the case was incurable at the outset. The remedy and dose failed to rouse the patient's vital force enough to provoke a curative response. Instead, it completely overwhelmed the severely weakened vital force; a curative response was impossible, and the whole organism turned to destruction. The selected dose was too high for the weakened state of the vital force and the medicine selected penetrated too deeply. This time, the error of judgement regarding remedy and dose selection occurred because the practitioner failed to perceive that destructive organic pathology was actually present rather than merely threatening.

> This kind of response is sometimes observed...in chronic, deep-seated disease as a result of the overreaction to a deeply acting antipsoric or antisyphilitic medicine, given in too high a potency at the beginning of treatment. If the potency is too high its action may be too deep and far-reaching, and the reaction too great for the weakened vital power to carry on...Very high potencies of the closely similar remedy are merciless searchers-out of hidden things. They will sometimes bring to light a veritable avalanche of symptoms, which overwhelm the

---

[179] Ibid

weakened patient. The disease has gone too far for such radical probing.[180]

Action:

The case must be handled with extreme care, as it is seldom that such patients recover perfectly.[181]

Follow guidelines given for the preceding unfavourable responses: *Prolonged intensification of original symptoms followed by gradual improvement,* and *Symptoms move in non-curative direction.*
To avoid making this mistake, when patients present in a doubtfully curable state due to insufficiency of prevailing vital force:

...Use medium potencies...and if necessary go higher gradually, as treatment progresses and the patient improves.[182]

Medium/moderate centesimal potencies mean 30c, 200c. Often, borderline doubtfully curable patients are made comfortable and respond very well to the LM/Q dosing regimen (see Chapter 11).

Original symptoms intensify followed by short interval of improvement then relapse

After taking the remedy, the chronically ill patient returns and reports 'I got worse for a while except for four or five days when I felt better, then I got much worse again.'

Evaluation:

The relapsing state may indicate:

...The remedy was only partly similar, or insufficient as to dosage; but where this occurrence is observed several times in succession and lasting improvement does not follow carefully selected remedies, it

---

[180] Dr. S. Close, *The Genius of Homœopathy*

[181] *Kent's New Remedies, Clinical Cases, Lesser Writings, Aphorisms and Precepts,* compiled by Dr. W.W. Sherwood

[182] Dr. S. Close, *The Genius of Homœopathy*

means that the case is incurable. There is not vitality enough to sustain a curative reaction, and dissolution is imminent.[183]

Action:

The seriousness of this situation dictates that utmost caution is taken. Calmly and methodically apply logic to the case analysis. The symptom-similarity between illness and remedy suitability must be improved. Review the original analysis, the basis of the prescription with the patient. Instruct the patient to correct any inaccuracies either in their descriptions or practitioner understanding. Review each characteristic symptom used in the hierarchy. When I am managing this obstacle in my own practice, I tell the patient: 'My original prescription basis needs more clarity. Please confirm that I have understood your suffering properly. Listen carefully as I go through each symptom and correct any errors I have made. If there is something that has been completely left out of this picture, especially if you think it is important, please let me know.' Restudy the case, and conduct a new case analysis. Select the remedy that more closely resembles patient's symptom totality of suffering.

If the symptom totality is unclear after the patient–practitioner review, and provided the patient is able to tolerate the condition, suspend treatment to await clarity. Wait watchfully, checking in with the patient at regular twice-weekly intervals. Watch and wait actively for a clearer symptom picture to emerge, which may indicate a different remedy is required.

If the review of the case indicates the same remedy as previously selected is still the most suitable, it may be repeated. Due to the complexity of the illness, the appropriate dosing method under consideration should be changed to the LM/Q dosing method, as this is the gentlest dosing method and ideal for relapsing states with severe pathology. According to LM/Q dosing protocols (see Chapter 11), the patient begins dosing and reports to the practitioner at three- to five-day intervals for progress assessment and dosing instructions.

---

[183] Dr. S. Close, *The Genius of Homœopathy*

Severe intensification of original symptoms plus development of organic pathology

After taking frequent repeated doses of a remedy in the lower 3c–24c potency range, the patient reports, or the practitioner observes, severe intensification of symptoms related to vital organ pathology, e.g. brain, lungs, heart, kidneys, etc.

Evaluation:

This unfavourable response to a well-chosen medicine indicates that the patient's vital force has overreacted to too frequent repetition of low potencies that did not match the proportion of strength with which the vital force prevailed in the patient. The non-curative response of the vital force might be so severe that it threatens the patient's life. This is especially harmful if the patient is a child or hypersensitive individual and the seat of the disturbance is in the brain or lungs. Dr. Close describes such an overreaction of the vital force in a case of 'meningitis', where low doses of Belladonna (3c or 6c) were given too frequently.

> The more accurate the selection of the medicine, the closer it is to the similimum, the greater must be the care exercised not to injure the patient by prescribing potencies too low and doses too numerous. [184]

> The careless prescriber rarely recognises such aggravations. When he notices the symptoms he usually attributes them to the natural course of disease or calls it a 'complication.'[185]

Action:

> On the first appearance of such aggravations, medication should be stopped immediately. If the aggravations do not speedily diminish, interrupt the response of the vital force with an antidote remedy that is known or a better-selected remedy should be administered.[186]

---

[184] Dr. S. Close, *The Genius of Homœopathy*

[185] Ibid.

[186] Ibid

Knowledgeable rapid intervention is required to manage this unfavourable response effectively. However, careless prescribers forget that effectiveness of homœopathy lies in the practitioner's knowledge of, and adherence to, Hahnemann's fixed fundamental principles of homœopathic practice. In this instance, see Chapter 1 Smallest Dose: dilution and potentiation, and the Proper Dose: Single Substance, Single Dose fixed principles. Lack of knowledge leads these prescribers to confuse signs of uninterrupted disease progress with a natural *brief* curative intensification of a patient's characteristic original symptoms.

Contending with non-curative complicated patient responses often makes us feel inadequate. In order to reduce patient suffering and correct flawed thinking, it is necessary to replace hubris with humility and seek urgent advice from a more experienced colleague. In that way, ignorance concerning effective management of potentially incurable cases is replaced with knowledge and the opportunity for a rapid curative response to be established increases.

Appearance of new symptoms

After taking the remedy the patient returns and reports: 'You cured me of the symptoms I had, but now I have new symptoms.'

Exercise caution. There are 5 possible evaluations:

1. The 'new' symptoms are not truly new
2. The practitioner administered a medicine whose true pure effects on the healthy were not perfectly known
3. In an acute illness, a frequently repeated remedy has accidentally produced 'new' medicinal symptoms
4. The patient has never experienced the 'new' symptoms before, they are troublesome, unrelated to the original illness and persist
5. The first remedy was imperfectly selected because its selection was based on *too few* symptoms

Possible Evaluation 1:

The 'new' symptoms are not truly new; they are long-forgotten symptoms resurfacing—previously unreported old original symptoms returning. The remedy was correctly chosen and the vital force is still responding curatively to it. The appearance of this type of 'new' symptom is manna from heaven to the practitioner because it confirms the accuracy of the remedy and dose selection.

Action:

To test this hypothesis, examine the patient carefully. If re-examination confirms the 'new' symptoms are not truly new, that they had been experienced before and forgotten, then the vital force is acting curatively in response to the remedy; it has brought back previously unresolved symptoms for final resolution. Everything is going according to plan. Therefore, do nothing except educate the patient regarding what has happened. WAIT for the remedy to cease influencing the vital force. A lull will follow the storm, the symptoms will gradually disappear and the patient will feel better.

Examine the patient to understand exactly when these forgotten symptoms appeared for the first time and amend the timeline accordingly. Add the so-called new symptoms to the original symptom totality list. At each subsequent progress report, review the status of all symptoms, including the 'new' ones. When the original symptoms rise up again to bother the patient, repeat the remedy that induced a curative response in a slightly modified dose.

Possible Evaluation 2:

The practitioner administered a medicine whose true pure effects on the healthy were not perfectly known. Only a portion of the symptoms of the illness could be healed by that medicine. The imperfect medicine was administered for lack of a more perfect one.[187] In this case we cannot expect a complete, undisturbed cure from this medicine; because during its use some symptoms appear that were not previously observable in the disease, accessory symptoms of the not perfectly appropriate remedy. This response does not prevent a considerable part of the disease (those symptoms of the disease that resemble those of the medicine administered) from being eradicated by that medicine and establishing a fair commencement of cure, but this cure does not take place without those accessory (new) symptoms, which are always moderate provided the dose of the medicine is sufficiently minute.[188]

This response usually happens where remedy selection is based upon uncharacteristic, indistinct, indefinite, common symptoms and vaguely described, general states: nausea, debility headache, and so forth.[189]

> Owing to the increased number of medicines whose pure effects are now known, such a case (administration of an inappropriate medicine) is *very rare*, and when they do occur, the bad effects resulting from it are diminished whenever a subsequent medicine of more accurate resemblance can be selected.[190]

Action:

In the treatment of chronic or acute illnesses, where the accessory symptoms are not severe, *wait* for the response of the vital force to stop and the accessory (new) symptoms to disappear.

Possible Evaluation 3:

In the treatment of *acute illness* where a remedy is repeated frequently, the 'new' symptoms may be symptoms that the correctly chosen medicine has the power to induce in healthy people, and the patient is experiencing them due to a high degree

---

[187] Dr. S. Hahnemann, *The Organon of Medicine*, Sixth edition, §162

[188] Ibid §163

[189] Ibid §165

[190] Ibid §166

of susceptibility or exceptional sensitivity to that particular medicine. Consequently, the 'new symptom' response indicates the patient is accidentally conducting a homœopathic drug trial/proving of that medicine. Left alone, these symptoms will gradually resolve without intervention. This type of 'new' symptom is usually trifling, rather than troublesome. Homœopathic patients report them because they consider them to be odd and have been educated to report all minor and major changes.

Action:

Check the 'new' symptoms in the homœopathic *Materia Medica* proving data related to the remedy administered. If they are listed, then that indicates that particular medicine has the power to artificially induce that symptom in healthy people. It confirms an accidental proving has occurred. Provided the symptom is mild and tolerable, WAIT watchfully. Report your findings to the patient. Explain that the reason for waiting is to allow the symptoms to disappear of their own accord.

If the 'new' symptoms are NOT found in the drug trial data, they may still disappear of their own volition. Therefore, it is still wise WAIT actively and not intervene before making another prescription.

If these 'new' symptoms persist and become intolerable for the patient, the appropriate strategy for managing the problem is described in **Action for Evaluation (4)** below.

Possible Evaluation 4:

Re-examination of the patient determines the patient has never experienced the 'new' symptoms before, they are troublesome, unrelated to the original illness and persist.

> Every medicine prescribed for a case of disease, which produces new and troublesome symptoms not appertaining to the disease to be cured, is not capable of effecting real improvement and cannot be considered as homœopathically selected.

Every aggravation by the production of new symptoms—when nothing untoward has occurred in the mental or physical regimen—invariably proves unsuitableness on the part of the medicine formerly given in the case of disease before us, but never indicates that the dose has been too weak.[191]

Action:

Therefore, if the aggravation is considerable, it must be partially neutralised by an antidote, before giving the next more accurately chosen symptom similar remedy.

If no antidote is known:

If the troublesome new symptoms be not very violent, the next remedy must be given immediately, in order to take the place of the improperly selected one.[192] The well informed and conscientiously careful physician will never require an antidote in his practice if, he will begin, as he should, with the selected medicine in the smallest possible dose. A similarly minute dose of a better chosen remedy will re-establish order throughout.[193]

Once again, reliable information regarding antidotal effects of remedies on one another is to be found in Hahnemann's *Materia Medica Pura* and *The Chronic Diseases: Their Peculiar Nature and Their Homœopathic Cure*. For example, in his preamble to the Pulsatilla medicine test[194] Hahnemann recommends:

When Pulsatilla has been given in too large a dose, or in an unsuitable case, and consequently it has produced disagreeable effects, according to their peculiar character, these may be removed by Chamomilla (particularly when drowsiness, exhaustion, and diminution of the senses are permanent), or by an infusion of coffee, (e.g. in the timorous anxiety), or by Ignatia or Nux Vomica. The fever, the disposition to weep, and the pains of Pulsatilla with all their after sufferings can be most quickly removed by the tincture of raw coffee.

---

[191] Dr. S. Hahnemann, *The Organon of Medicine*, Sixth edition §249

[192] Ibid

[193] Ibid

[194] Dr. S. Hahnemann, *Materia Medica Pura*

The phrase 'according to their peculiar character' is extremely significant. It means these remedies should never be applied routinely in all instances of overreaction to Pulsatilla; that selection of one of these remedies should only be made where the symptom-similarity totality agrees, i.e. if the characteristic disagreeable symptoms experienced are similar to the characteristic symptoms artificially induced in healthy people by *Chamomilla*, or *Ignatia*, or *Nux Vomica*.

To identify a more suitable homœopathic remedy, review the illness history for lack and inaccuracy of information. With the patient's help, fill information gaps and correct any errors, reanalyse the state and select a remedy that resembles the original illness more closely than the previous one.

> Any subsequent prescription takes into account all the things that have preceded it, all the conditions that have arisen, and, the third, fourth, fifth or Sixth prescriptions have the same difficulties to surmount. If the first prescription was an unfortunate one, then all the others are made with difficulty and fear.[195]

Possible Evaluation 5:

The appearance of 'new' symptoms may also indicate the first remedy was imperfectly selected because its selection was based on *too few* symptoms. The practitioner perceived only part of the symptom totality rather than the complete, whole-symptom totality; one side of illness rather than the whole illness.

According to Hahnemann[196] the imperfect selection of the medicine is most commonly caused by too few symptoms of the illness being discovered, none that accurately resemble the distinctive (characteristic) peculiar, uncommon symptoms of the case of disease.

The only diseases that seem to have too few symptoms are those that may be termed one-sided diseases because they display only one or two principal or severe, violent symptoms that seem to

---

[195] Dr. J. T. Kent, *Lectures on Homœopathic Philosophy*

[196] Dr. S. Hahnemann, *The Organon of Medicine*, Sixth edition, §162–§208

obscure almost all the others. They belong chiefly to the class of chronic diseases.

Their principal symptom may be either an internal complaint (e.g. a headache of many years' duration, a diarrhoea of long standing, and ancient cardialgia, etc.) or it may be an affection of a more external local kind.

Often, *one-sided* diseases consisting of only an internal complaint are to be attributed to the practitioner's lack of ability to judge that all the symptoms really present have been discovered.[197]

> ...The oftener you prescribe for different groups of symptoms the worse it is for your patient, because it tends to rivet the constitutional state upon the patient and make him incurable. Do not prescribe until you have found the remedy that is similar to the whole case, even although it is clear in your mind that one remedy may be more similar to one particular group of symptoms and another remedy to another group.[198]

Action:

> Reexamine the patient to enable completion of the disease portrait sketch.[199]

Practitioners who are aware that their original patient examination elicited only a portion of the symptom image totality —and have re-examined the patient but still discover only a portion of the illness rather than the totality—understand that to avoid unnecessary complications and suffering, it is very wise to select each dose with great caution. For this important reason: administration of imperfectly selected remedies often induces new *'accessory symptoms'* and complications such as those described below.

During the use of imperfectly selected not homœopathic remedies, some symptoms appear that were not previously observable, accessory symptoms of the imperfectly selected

---

[197] Ibid

[198] Dr. J. T.Kent, *Lectures on Homœopathic Philosophy*

[199] Dr. S. Hahnemann, *The Organon of Medicine*, Sixth edition §175

remedy, which are mixed up with the patient's state of health; or symptoms appear that the patient had never previously experienced; or others that were previously only felt indistinctly become more pronounced.[200] Provided the appearance of these accessory symptoms was not caused by an important error in way of life or diet, a violent emotion, or a tumultuous revolution in the organism such as the occurrence or cessation of the menstrual flow, conception, childbirth, etc., the accessory symptoms and new symptoms that appear were induced by the medicine given, owing to its power to cause similar symptoms. [201]

To simplify this complicated situation, provided the patient is able to tolerate these 'accessory' symptoms, wait and watch, allow them to resolve naturally without intervention. Exercising caution when selecting each dose pays dividends. Hahnemann says: accessory symptoms always tend to be moderate when the dose of medicine is sufficiently minute.[202]

However, watching and waiting for nature to resolve the situation is not an option in treatment of *acute*, urgent care illnesses, where the patient's state is rapidly growing perceptibly worse hour to hour.

Hahnemann says: during the use of this imperfectly homœopathic remedy, if accessory symptoms of some strength occur, then in treatment of an *acute illnesses* we do not allow this first dose to exhaust its action. We investigate the morbid state afresh, in the now altered condition, and in tracing a new picture of the disease add the remainder of original symptoms to those newly developed. [203] We shall then be able to more readily discover a more suitable symptom-similar medicine, a single dose of which, if it does not destroy the original disease, will considerably advance it towards cure.

---

[200] Ibid §180

[201] Ibid §181

[202] Ibid §163

[203] Ibid §167

And thus we go on, if even this medicine is not quite sufficient to effect the restoration of health, examining again and again the morbid state that still remains, and selecting a homœopathic medicine as suitable as possible for it, until our objective of putting the patient in the possession of perfect health is accomplished.[204]

Thus the imperfect selection of the medicament, which was in this case almost inevitable owing to the existence of *too few symptoms*, serves to complete the display of the illness symptoms and facilitates discovery of a second more accurately suitable, homœopathic medicine.[205]

With Hahnemann, the devil is always in the detail. These particular instructions, which refer to the treatment of *acute* diseases, are often unintentionally misapplied to the treatment of chronic illness. This leads to changing of remedies every time the chronic condition changes. It spoils excellent prescriptions, creates a great muddle and induces avoidable extra suffering.

Experience of unfavourable vital force responses tests patients' patience! During this time, you work swiftly to correct errors, reduce anxiety by honestly and openly discussing what happened with the patient. In the midst of unravelling a muddle, Dr. Kent's invaluable advice assuages practitioner fear and aids concentration:

The patient will wait better if the doctor confesses on the spot that the selection was not what it ought to be, and he hopes to do better next time. It is a strange thing how patients will have an increase of confidence if the doctor will tell the truth. The acknowledgement of one's own ignorance begets confidence in an intelligent patient.[206]

The confidence of the patient helps the physician to find the right remedy. His mind works much better when he feels he is trusted; the confidence of the patient sharpens his intelligence.[207]

---

[204] Ibid §168

[205] Ibid §182

[206] Dr. J.T. Kent, *Lectures on Homœopathic Philosophy*

[207] Ibid

Evaluation of vital force responses to the homœopathic medicine, demands logic-rooted practitioner intelligence. To avoid confusion and unnecessary additional patient suffering it is wise to heed the axiom 'More haste, less speed'.

The next chapter describes vital force curative and non-curative responses to LM/Q potency dosage.

11

LM/Q Potency Response Analysis

At the beginning of treatment using LM/Q doses, frequent patient assessment by phone is required to ensure each patient receives the correct dose at proper intervals, and that necessary adjustments are made promptly. A common practitioner obstacle is feeling overwhelmed and confused by receiving too much information, too frequently. When using LM/Q potencies, this is especially so in the treatment of chronic illness, rather than urgent care illness. To avoid that serious obstacle to recovery, *before the patient starts dosing,* the practitioner prepares a mini symptom totality portrait for comparison purposes. It consists of a few (maximum six) extremely significant, distinctive characteristic features and individualising symptoms that represent the patient's illness. Where relevant, the ideal mini symptom totality portrait includes one characteristic symptom for each of the following spheres of suffering:

- Mental and emotional
- The degree of energy measured according to the 0–10 scale, where zero equals no energy, and ten equals high energy

- A discharge from a normal channel, orifice, pustule, vesicle, blister or wound, e.g. tears, perspiration, blood, mucous, pus, sputum, vomit, diarrhoea, urine, etc.
- Sleep disturbance pattern
- The most afflicted region of the body

Due to the small amount of illness information under review, each brief five- or seven-day interval progress report and assessment should take less than ten minutes: five minutes to collect the information, two minutes to consider the correct action plan and three minutes to explain it to the patient.

Depending on whether the patient improves or worsens, the patient will be instructed to continue, stop or resume dosing at each of these reports.

At the end of the first month, it is common for intelligent patients to become familiar with signs indicating when dosing should be stopped and that they should call the practitioner for further instructions.

At the beginning of LM/Q dosing, be prepared for patient lack of complicance and resistance to reporting frequently. This is especially likely from: individuals who dislike being what they consider to be 'micro-managed'; those who are extremely worried about their condition, or people who are highly sensitive and unable to think clearly about what they are doing. At first, these individuals may experience significant difficulty with the LM/Q dosing method. Following instructions is difficult for them. They may make up the medicine dose incorrectly, take the medicine too frequently, or forget to take it all. Practitioner calmness, patience, perseverance, encouragement and reassurance are particularly essential here to guide patients forward and correct any dosing errors. Extra time spent educating patients in the short term pays dividends in the long-term. In my own practice, the instructions are written out and we read them through together for clarity. Dosing does not begin until I am confident they have been understood properly.

Even so, things may go wrong. At the end of the first month, if the patient's actions indicate absolute inability to follow practitioner directions, switching to the centesimal dosing method and its own attendant difficulties may be the only remaining option. Before deciding to make that switch, discuss the option thoroughly with the patient, especially the typical increased potential for overreactions and other case management problems that may arise. If a switch to centesimal dosing is made, to ensure minimal disruption to the vital force always start with a moderate dose (e.g. 30c) and ascend the scale over time.

If LM/Q dosing continues smoothly, and once the practitioner is confident that the individual understands when to call for evaluation and instructions, the seven-day interval reports may be replaced with brief reports on an as-needed basis. More comprehensive reports should occur at regular four to five weekly intervals.

When using the LM/Q dosing method in the treatment of longstanding illness, the rule is to commence homœopathic treatment with the smallest possible doses and only gradually increase their power by a thorough, vigorous shaking of the bottle before administration of the medicine once daily.[208]

That rule is subject to a notable exception in the homœopathic treatment of inherited predisposition related skin conditions— before local old school treatment has been instituted—where external signs of the inner predispositions burst forth and remain in full view and the patient does not suffer any concurrent internal symptoms. Examples of these include a recently erupted itching skin condition indicating the presence of Psora, or the untouched chancre (on the sexual organs, labia, mouth or lips, and so forth) indicating the presence of the Syphilitic predisposition, or the fig warts, indicating the presence of the Sycotic predisposition. These particular skin conditions have not yet been treated; therefore, they not only tolerate, they also require large doses of their symptom-similar remedies in ever higher and higher potency (possibly also several times daily).[209]

---

[208] Dr. S. Hahnemann, *The Organon of Medicine*, Sixth edition §247,

[209] Ibid, §282 F/n 163

It is significant that Hahnemann recommends increasing LM/ Q dosing frequency to more than once daily only for a very specific set of circumstances. He warns: such treatment of diseases hidden within would be dangerous, because while the excessive dose extinguishes the disease, its continued usage initiates, possibly produces a medicinal disease, making the patient worse.[210] As a rule, too large doses of an accurately chosen homœopathic medicine, especially when frequently repeated, causes much trouble. They put the patient's life in danger or make his disease almost incurable.[211]

The LM/Q potency progress examination compares the patient's state before and after receiving the remedy in the context of the natural direction of cure. This is to assess whether patient and illness are moving in the curative and correct, rather than the non-curative, incorrect direction. Once again the instruments for comparison are: (a) original illness Totality of Characteristic Individualising Symptoms, and (b) the Birth to Present Timeline that reflects the order in which each symptom or condition first appeared.

Within the different recovery timeframes (i.e. shorter in urgent care, and longer for chronic illness), a *positive* curative response is signalled by the original *existing* symptoms moving centrifugally outward from within. Simultaneously, the patient's energy increases and mental and emotional symptoms decrease or disappear first. Next, physical discomfort decreases from the top downward: from head to hand to toe; from most important organ[s] to least important organ[s]. Often all symptoms disappear in the reverse chronological order in which they appeared. (See discussion in Chapter 7)

> ...When these symptoms of the illness go from center to circumference, going out from the centers of life, out from the heart, lungs, brain and spine, out from the interiors onto the extremities, it is

---

[210] Ibid, §282 F/n 163

[211] Ibid §276

well...Eruptions on the skin and affections in the extremities are good signs.[212]

Should information gleaned indicate the opposite has occurred —for example where before treatment a patient suffered psychological and skin troubles, and in response to the remedy the skin symptoms improve and the psychological suffering worsens— that response indicates that the illness has moved from a less important organ to a more important organ, and the patient is moving in the non-curative, wrong direction.

The non-curative response to the remedy must be interrupted; the original symptom image totality must be reviewed, information already given needs to be clarified, expanded and confirmed, new information sought and earlier analysis errors identified and corrected. In the corrected reanalysis, a new, more suitable remedy may appear for selection and administration, one that will interrupt the negative response to the previous remedy.

Concerning rhythms of response to homœopathic medicines and what Hahnemann describes as the 'so-called' homœopathic aggravation, major differences between centesimal and LM/Q dosing methods exist. After ingestion of a centesimal dose, a curative response is understood to have occurred when—within minutes in acute disease or one hour to ten days in chronic disease —a patient may experience a brief slight intensification of original symptoms that is always followed rapidly by lasting improvement. In other words, the intensification occurs soon after ingesting the medicine. In LM/Q potency dosing, the reverse is true.

As a rule, in response to daily LM/Q doses of a well-chosen remedy, patients begin to improve immediately. After the patient has experienced continued improvement for some time, the intensification of original symptoms occurs, indicating the vital force has received slightly more medicine than it needed and it is feeling over-stimulated. The patient is directed to stop LM/Q dosing for a while. Within minutes or a few hours, that original symptom intensification rapidly disappears. Without medicine, the

---

[212] Dr. J. T. Kent, *Lectures on Homœopathic Philosophy*

patient resumes improvement experienced before the intensification. There is no need for another dose of medicine until the return of original symptoms signals that the vital force is calling for more assistance, at which time the patient resumes LM/Q dosing from the point in the Stock Bottle where they left off.

LM/Q potency responses tend to fall into these categories:

- Patient and symptoms improve *without* intensification of original symptoms
- Disappearance of *some* original symptoms and increase of other original symptoms
- Original symptoms improve continuously then reappearance of original symptoms
- Patient discontinues dosing and original symptoms persist
- Mental, emotional symptoms worsen while physical symptoms improve
- Original symptoms intensify immediately after patient starts LM/Q dosing regimen
- Uncomfortable changes to original symptoms occur and new symptoms appear
- Lack of reaction

Patient and symptoms improve *without* intensification of original symptoms

The patient begins taking the remedy, once daily. At the first seven-day brief check-in, the patient reports: 'I am feeling much better, the symptoms I had have disappeared and nothing new has come up.'

Evaluation:
The remedy is affecting the patient's vital force curatively.

Action:
So long as the patient experiences continued improvement, and does not experience one or another complaint that he

never had before in his life i.e. new symptoms, the patient continues to dose daily or every second day.[213]

Provided the patient continues to improve steadily without experiencing new symptoms, consideration may be given at the fourth seven-day interval brief report to extending the interval between reports to once every ten to fourteen days, while *still continuing* the comprehensive progress report at four weekly intervals.

Disappearance of *some* original symptoms but increase of other original symptoms

'I've been taking the remedy every day and quite a few of my symptoms have gone away, but the ones that are left have become a little worse.'

Evaluation:

During daily repetition of the well-indicated homœopathic remedy, many symptoms of the original natural illness disappear, but the balance (remainder) of symptoms seem to increase. This response indicates the patient has received an excess of medicine, the symptom-similar artificial medicinal disease alone exists and persistently manifests itself.[214]

Action:

In this situation, to know if any more medicine is required and how much, each dose must be reduced further and repeated at longer intervals or possibly stopped for several days, to see if the symptoms disappear by themselves.[215]

When faced with more than one action option, it is wise to try each action option separately, and in turn, and assess the patient's

---

[213] Dr. S. Hahnemann, *The Organon of Medicine*, Sixth edition, §248

[214] Ibid §248

[215] Ibid §248

response to each action option in, for example, seven days to gain clarity regarding the correct action. If that action does not induce improvement, try the next option. If the first two action options are tried and improvement does not occur, stop dosing:

> If the apparent increase of symptoms is the result of excess medicine, they will soon disappear and leave undisturbed health in its wake.

> If after stopping the medicine for a certain period of eight, ten or fifteen days, traces of the original symptoms reappear, they are remnants of the original disease, not completely extinguished and must be treated with higher potencies of the same medicine, as directed before. The patient resumes dosing where they left off.[216]

Original symptoms improve continuously then some original symptoms reappear in mild to moderate degree of intensity

'I started feeling better—almost as soon as I began taking the medicine, right away, mentally physically and emotionally. Today a few of my old symptoms have come back. Some of them bother me a bit, others bother me a lot, but not as much as they did before.'

Evaluation:

The patient started daily dosing. As directed, the patient modified every dose, gradually moving up the potency scale: LM/Q#01, then LM/Q#02, LM/Q#03 and so on. All went well. Then, while their overall feeling is generally improved, the patient begins to experience the return of one or more of the *original* symptoms, which reappear in a mild to moderate degree.

The reappearance of *original* symptoms indicates that the artificial disease of the homœopathic medicine, which is very similar to the natural disease, is now the only one influencing the vital force; this suggests recovery may be imminent. Reinvigorated, the vital force has almost no more need of the assistance provided

---

[216] Ibid §281

by the remedy. Free of the natural disease, the vital force is beginning to suffer somewhat from an excess of the homœopathic medicine. The patient is now experiencing the so-called 'homœopathic aggravation', as it were, at the end of treatment.[217]

Action:

To confirm that recovery is imminent, the patient discontinues dosing for seven to fourteen days. During this interval off the medicine, if the reappearing symptoms are those of the artificial medicinal disease they will disappear within a few hours or days, leaving unclouded health in their wake. Provided the patient continues the recommended lifestyle changes, no more symptoms will manifest, and the patient will probably be cured.[218]

If the reappearing symptoms continue during the interval off the remedy, the patient is experiencing vital force response three, which is discussed next.

Patient discontinues dosing and original symptoms persist

'I'm calling because I have been off the remedy for ten days. You told me the symptoms that came back before I stopped dosing would go away, but they haven't.'

Evaluation:

At the end of a period without medicine, remnants of the previously observed (original) disease still manifest.[219] This response indicates that the original disease has not yet been completely extinguished. Traces of the original complaint remain.

---

[217] Dr. S. Hahnemann, *The Organon of Medicine*, Sixth edition, §146, §248, §280

[218] Ibid §248, §281

[219] Ibid §281

Action:

In order to advance the patient toward cure, treatment with higher potencies must be renewed.[220] Dosing should be resumed from the point in the Stock Bottle where the patient left off, and at the same intervals as previously.

Patients who receive the correct symptom-similar homœopathic medicine and use the LM/Q dosing method tend to move rhythmically along the road to recovery something like this:

1. The patient starts dosing and original illness symptoms disappear
2. So long as the patient continues improving, they continue dosing. Then there is a return and intensification of original symptoms and the patient worsens, indicating that the patient has received too much medicine and the patient stops dosing
3. Off the medicine, the patient improves and, for a while, no more medicine is required
4. Then gradually, or suddenly, the original symptoms of the illness reappear, indicating the vital force is calling for more remedy
5. The patient resumes dosing from the point in the Stock Bottle where they left off, at the same frequency as before; the symptoms disappear again, so as long as the patient improves they dosing.
6. Then the original symptoms reappear, the patient stops dosing and the cycle begins again.

The further along the road to recovery the patient moves, and the closer to complete cure the patient gets, the less medicine the vital force needs and the quicker the patient reaches excess medicine. The sooner the patient stops dosing, the longer intervals the patient spends *off* the remedy free of symptoms.

Non-curative responses to LM/Q doses tend to fall into these categories:

---

[220] Ibid, §281

- Mental emotional symptoms worsen while physical symptoms improve
- Original symptoms intensify immediately at start of LM/Q dosing regimen
- Appearance of troublesome new and altered symptoms
- Lack of reaction

Mental emotional symptoms worsen while physical symptoms improve

'Before I started treatment, I felt awful mentally and emotionally. I was a wreck; my skin was in terrible shape. That's cleared up, but psychologically I am worse than ever.'

Evaluation:

Such a response signals the illness is moving in the non-curative, wrong direction—from the less important organ (skin) to a more important organ (brain). The remedy administered is incorrect. It was either completely incorrect or it is partially incorrect. It suited the outer regions of the person, but not the inner regions.

Action:

The patient stops dosing. The practitioner schedules daily reports to confirm that, off the remedy, the mental symptoms improve, and the patient begins to feel better.

Once the patient starts to feel better, *do not repeat* the remedy. Wait for the original symptom totality to re-emerge.

Meanwhile, urgently restudy the case from the beginning. To avoid repeating the same mistake, review the original history of the illness with the patient—all the characteristic individualising symptoms used as the prescription basis—to ensure nothing has been omitted or forgotten. Ask the patient to correct any errors. In that way, an improved, more complete symptom image totality will form the basis of the next prescription, compared to only a portion, and a remedy will be found that resembles the illness more closely.

Consult the homœopathic *Materia Medica* to confirm symptom-similarity accuracy of the newly chosen remedy. Once the practitioner is convinced the new remedy resembles the illness more closely, it may be administered in the LM/Q potency. As before, start at the beginning of the potency scale: LM/Q#01, dosing once daily. The patient should be monitored for changes at seven-day intervals. If improvement occurs, dosing is continued until the patient worsens, when dosing will stop.

Original symptoms intensify immediately at start of LM/Q dosing regimen

After the first LM/Q dose, the patient experiences a marked intensification of all the original symptoms of the illness. 'I know I've only had one dose but I feel dreadful, much worse. All the symptoms I have are much worse in every way, so I had to call you.'

Evaluation:

After the first LM/Q dose, the patient experiences a marked intensification of the original symptoms of the illness. There are two likely probabilities:

- The remedy was correct but the dose was too strong
- The remedy was incorrectly selected

Either way the intensification of symptoms must be reduced.

Action:

To test if the response was 'a sure sign that, although the remedy was correct, the doses were altogether too large',[221] reduce the strength of the dose by modifying it according to the rules applied to managing overreactions experienced by unusually excited and sensitive individuals:

---

[221] Dr. S. Hahnemann, *The Organon of Medicine*, Sixth edition, §282

...A *teaspoonful* of the first glass may be put in a second glass of 7–8 tablespoons of water, thoroughly stirred and *teaspoonful* doses be given. There are patients of so great sensitivity that a third or fourth glass similarly prepared may be necessary.[222]

Always review the patient's state at seven-day intervals.

In pediatric and veterinary homœopathic medicine, infants and animals are unable to describe their suffering. This presents practitioners with the obstacle of paucity of information gathered during the patient examination. This lack of information increases the potential for imperfect selection of medicines. That being true, to avoid changing medicines too early and risk spoiling the case, it is wiser to first reduce the dose as described and wait watchfully for any signs of improvement.

Whether patients are human or animal, to ensure clarity of response assessment, it is always extremely wise to be systematic and avoid intermingling dose modifications. For example, if the dose modification is volume dilution from first glass to second glass, etc., let the patient stay with that particular glass dilution for seven days and then evaluate them before altering the dose. After reassessing, if necessary, go to third glass dilution for a week. If this doesn't work, go to the fourth glass dilution. However, it is vitally important that you reassess at the end of each week before altering the dose. If the modification selected is tablespoonful to teaspoonful volume dilution, the patient should stay with that dosing regimen for seven days and then be reassessed.

If the dose modification selected is extending intervals between doses, try once every other day for a week and reassess, then, if necessary, once every two days for a week and reassess, and so on, gradually extending the intervals between doses and reassessment to once every seven days.

If, after the dose has been modified by dilutions and intervals between doses, the original symptoms persist or intensify, such a response indicates the remedy selected is very likely incorrect.

---

[222] Ibid §248

Discontinue dosing. Restudy the case thoroughly from the beginning, identify and correct analysis mistakes, select a more suitable medicine that more accurately reflects the symptom totality and administer it.

After re-examining the patient and restudying the case, if the same remedy is indicated, it cannot be given again as it has not induced a curative response from the vital force. There is nothing that can be done now, but wait for a change in the suffering, for some new, never-had-before symptom to appear. This new symptom can be added to the original symptom totality and may then lead to another medicine , one with greater symptom-similarity to the suffering experienced. While waiting for the change in suffering to emerge, it is valuable to consider the possibility of the existence of an undetected maintaining cause and examine the patient accordingly. To confirm or deny the presence of a constraining maintaining cause, follow the relevant guidance offered below in the section *Lack of Reaction; second probability*.

Uncomfortable changes to original symptoms occur and new symptoms appear

'I've been dosing daily and something has come up that I've never had before at all, and most of the other symptoms feel as though they changed and they're bothering me a lot.'

Evaluation:

A medicine that during its action on the vital force, produces new and troublesome symptoms not appertaining to the original disease to be cured, is not capable of effecting real improvement and cannot be considered homœopathically selected.[223]

If the new, altered symptoms came and went without troubling the patient, no intervention would be required. It is the troublesome, persisting nature of these new altered symptoms that

---

[223] Dr. S. Hahnemann, *The Organon of Medicine*, Sixth edition, §249

indicates the need to intervene. A significant change in the nature of the original illness has occurred and the original symptom totality may have shifted into an entirely new state. To continue towards permanent recovery, the vital force may require a different symptom-similar remedy—a more homœopathically related medicine, one that has the power to induce symptoms that more closely resemble those of the new and significantly altered state. [224]

Action:

The patient stops dosing.

To avoid changing remedies inappropriately, the practitioner examines the patient carefully to confirm that the new altered symptoms have truly never been experienced before, rather than being a reappearance of something previously forgotten and not reported.

After confirming the symptoms have never been experienced before, it is safe to conclude a new state has emerged requiring a change of remedy. The practitioner reanalyses the case using the previous original symptom image totality and expands it to include the persisting troublesome *new and altered* symptoms that indicate the emergence of a new state.

> ...Administer the new remedy in the same repeated doses, mindful before each dose to gradually modify and increase its potency with thorough, vigorous succussions.[225]

After administering the new remedy, to ensure necessary adjustments are made promptly, seven-day interval mini progress reports should be scheduled.

---

[224] Ibid §248

[225] Ibid §248 – §250

Lack of reaction

'It's seven days and nothing's changed. My physical energy is down, everything is the same as it was before I started treatment. What's going on?'

Evaluation:

The vital force appears not to have responded to the medicine. Existing original suffering has neither improved nor worsened. In this case, the two most likely probabilities to consider are:

- The remedy was incorrectly selected, and so the vital force did not respond
- A powerful maintaining cause of disease persists, preventing the vital force from responding.

Possible Evaluation 1: Incorrect remedy selection:

...When no improvement...ensues...it invariably proves unsuitability of the medicine formerly given for the case of disease before us...but never indicates that the dose has been too weak.[226]

Action:
Discontinue dosing.

...When no improvement ensues, we should act injudiciously and hurtfully were we *to repeat* or even *increase the dose* of the same medicine, as is done in the old system, under the delusion that it was not efficacious because of its small quantity (it's too small dose).[227]

Examine the patient respectfully and meticulously. The examination will either confirm the vital force did not respond at all in any way, shape or form—nothing untoward occurred to affect the prescribed course of treatment, e.g. the patient's mental and physical state, diet, way of life, etc.— or it will gently reveal something unexpected or self-inflicted (e.g. overwork, physical strain, injury) has occurred in the mental or physical regimen to

---

[226] Ibid §249, F/n 135

[227] Ibid

disrupt the response. Patient education usually removes such obstacles without the need for medication.

If the patient confidently confirms that none of the symptoms experienced before the remedy was ingested have changed in any way—even minutely—and no new symptoms have appeared, it is safe to conclude that vital force lack of reaction to the remedy has occurred because the remedy was incorrectly chosen.

In this situation, the search must continue for a different homœopathic remedy, one with greater symptom-similarity to the symptom image totality.

The practitioner restudies the case for errors in the symptom totality that was used as the basis of the previous prescription. The information is carefully reviewed with the patient to confirm its accuracy; any errors are corrected and any new information is included. Then the practitioner reanalyses the case from the beginning, consults the *Materia Medica* to confirm the remedy selection more accurately reflects the totality of suffering and selects a different remedy.

The new remedy is administered using the LM/Q dosing method, starting again at LM/Q#01 and ascending the potency scale. Doses are repeated once at daily intervals as before and the patient is monitored for changes at seven-day intervals.

Possible Evaluation 2: A powerful maintaining cause of disease persists

The second probability for a lack of reaction is there is a powerful maintaining cause of disease persisting *and* the patient's vital force has insufficient strength to contend with it. Hahnemann says:

But should we find, during the employment of the other medicines in chronic (psoric) diseases, that the best selected homœopathic (antipsoric) medicine in the suitable (minutest) dose does not effect an improvement, this is a *sure* sign that the cause that keeps up the disease still persists, and that there is some circumstance in the mode of life of the patient, or in the situation in which the patient is placed, that must be removed in order that a permanent cure may ensue. [228]

There could be several reasons for this 'maintaining cause': it was correctly identified as an obstacle to recovery at the outset of treatment and, although strategies for its removal were discussed and agreed with the patient, for some reason those strategies were not implemented, leaving the obstacle in place. Alternatively, at the time of the history-taking consultation, the maintaining cause may not have been revealed or identified, and so obstacle removal strategies were never discussed. The final reason is that the powerful maintaining cause has only recently emerged.

Action: Discontinue dosing.

That maintaining circumstance or situation must be removed to allow the vital force to respond and movement towards recovery may begin. Do not consider changing the remedy yet. Sensitively, examine the patient concerning the possible existence and nature of the maintaining cause. Discuss the need to free the vital force from the ball-and-chain effect of the maintaining cause. Some maintaining causes are life-long. In itself, consideration of their removal may prove to be daunting. Avoid the common desire to hasten the patient towards acting before they are ready to do so. The only way an obstacle may be removed is if the patient recognises its existence, consents to its removal and has the will to try to remove it. Ongoing practitioner encouragement should be offered. Collaborate with the patient to develop appropriate strategies to minimise and eliminate the constraining influence of the maintaining cause. Wait as long as is necessary until the patient feels comfortable and satisfied they possess sufficient courage to move against the obstacle.

When the patient confirms they are ready, instruct the patient to implement the strategies that have been discussed and agreed upon for not less than one month.

---

[228] Ibid §252

At one month, re-examine the patient to confirm that strategies have been implemented and the powerful influence of the maintaining cause has been minimised or removed.

If the lack of reaction was due to a maintaining cause, implementing obstacle removal strategies and leaving the patient without medicine for not less than one month provides an opportunity for some of the original symptoms to gradually disappear or their intensity to reduce. Where improvement occurs while the patient has stopped dosing, the strength of the vital force is understood to have improved. So long as improvement continues, the patient remains without medicine and is monitored for changes at regular intervals.

During this time, the practitioner is wise to review the basis of the prescription administered, ensure all information gathered is correct and the remedy already selected remains the most suitable for the illness experienced.

When the original symptoms reappear, the vital force is calling for more assistance. Provided the remedy already administered has been reconfirmed regarding its symptom-similarity suitability, the patient resumes dosing at the point in the Stock Bottle where dosing stopped and is monitored for progress and changes at seven-day intervals.

If the maintaining cause is removed, the patient is not dosing and there is still no improvement in the patient's energy or symptoms, the vital force needs help.

To determine the need to change remedies, it is necessary to prove that the remedy already selected is still unsuitable. The only way to do that is to instruct the patient to resume LM/Q dosing at the point in the Stock Bottle where dosing stopped. To ensure any further suffering is promptly curtailed, the patient must be monitored at three-day intervals or more frequently. If improvement ensues the patient continues dosing. If the patient worsens, the remedy is deemed to be unsuitable and dosing is discontinued.

The practitioner searches for a more suitable remedy and reviews information gathered so far with the patient, confirming its accuracy. Any information gaps or errors are filled and corrected. No stone is left unturned. The symptom image totality used as the basis for the previous prescription is reviewed. Reassured by the patient that everything about the suffering has been accurately understood, the practitioner reanalyses the case from the beginning, consults the *Materia Medica*, and selects a different remedy, one that more accurately reflects the totality of suffering.

The new remedy is administered using the LM/Q dosing method, starting again at LM/Q#01 and ascending the potency scale. Doses are repeated once at daily intervals as before and seven-day interval short reports should be scheduled to monitor the patient for changes. Information is gathered, reviewed and appropriate actions taken promptly.

After ingesting the new remedy, if the patient still does not respond to the apparently well-indicated remedy, there is either an undiscovered error in the practitioner's understanding of the case, or the patient may be incurable.

Discontinue dosing.

At this point in treatment, practitioner desperation usually sets in. Perseverance and humility are in high demand. The only way the practitioner may effectively eliminate the possibility of an undiscovered error is to diligently perform yet another thorough case review.

To avoid continued confusion and gain sufficient clarity, the practitioner's intellect must be refreshed. Consider applying adjunctive non-medicinal measures to relieve the worst of the discomfort. Put aside the case for a day or two and then tackle it again in the normal way. Always explain the proposed action plan to the patient to ensure they know what you are doing and why. That way the patient is less likely to feel cast adrift while waiting for the practitioner to complete the thinking process.

If patient re-examination and case reanalysis do not reveal a different remedy, resist the temptation to give a treatment that may be incorrect in the delusion that doing something is better than doing nothing. Such acts of desperation result in serious complications for the patient. It is wiser to leave the patient without medicine for some time while monitoring the patient closely for changes. Left alone, the vital force may produce more symptoms, at last guiding the practitioner to a more suitable remedy.

Where a maintaining cause cannot be removed and continues to constrain the vital force, patient and practitioner expectations regarding complete health restoration require adjustment. Due to insufficient strength with which the vital force prevails in the patient, permanent recovery may not be possible.

LM/Q dosing requires a high level of practitioner intelligence and proficiency, patient–practitioner collaboration and patient compliance. Compared to the centesimal preparation and dosing method, the LM/Q potency preparation is more refined, rendering the medicine even more accessible to the vital force. Most importantly, the LM/Q potency does exactly what Hahnemann intended: it moves patients faster along the road to recovery with less intense and shorter overreactions if any, it induces fewer response variations, and simplifies and improves progress assessment accuracy.

12

Changing Medicines

Ineffective homœopathy is most often due to prescribers improperly changing medicines. Usually this major mistake and obstacle to cure happens where a patient improves after the first dose, and that improvement includes a slight change in the existing symptoms without the appearance of any new symptoms. The practitioner thinks that a slight shift of symptoms always indicates the vital force is calling for a different of remedy. A new remedy and dose is selected, the improvement achieved earlier is brought to a halt and trouble begins. Then the prescriber gets rattled, doubtful and hurried. Attempting to interrupt a worsening situation, more and more remedy changes are made, and yet the patient is still sick.[229]

It is important to understand that a different remedy is *not* indicated:

- So long as the patient's mental and emotional disposition improves, physical energy increases, original symptoms disappear and reappear less intensely
- When a single symptom changes
- With each shift of symptoms

---

[229] Dr. S. Close, *The Genius of Homœopathy; Kent's new Remedies Clinical Cases Lesser Writings Aphorisms and Precepts*, compiled by Dr. W.W. Sherwood

- When symptoms change only slightly
- When the symptom image is in the process of changing

The proper time to ponder the question of whether the vital force has stopped responding to the current remedy and is calling for a different remedy to continue recovery is when **all** the following factors are present at the same time: *persisting, multiple, pronounced, new, never experienced before, very bothersome symptoms.*

Careless, rapid, improper changes of remedies create complex muddles and avoidable patient suffering. While advising practitioners struggling with problematic cases, I have observed so many different remedies have been prescribed—in various potencies and improperly repeated—that the original, once sharp and colourful portrait of the illness blurs beyond recognition. Regrettably, the only way to unscramble such confusion and regain a moderate degree of clarity is to leave the patient's bruised and battered vital force alone without medicine, using non-medicinal adjunctive measures to ease the discomfort, while carefully monitoring the patient for changes, even though implementing that case managemetn strategy means that the patient suffers terribly. During the hiatus, if the patient does not opt to discontinue homœopathic treatment in disgust, and providing the prevailing strength of the vital force has not been irreparably weakened by the practitioner's hasty actions, the vital force may eventually rally and reproduce the original symptom image. If that happens, the practitioner should thank their lucky stars, reanalyse the case very carefully, select a more suitable symptom-similar medicine and administer it in a moderate dose. In this situation, the safest dosing method for consideration would be the most gentle: the LM/Q dosing method accompanied by frequent patient monitoring.

Golden rules for changing medicines

In the homœopathic treatment of long-term illness, Hahnemann advises practitioners to allow all remedies to act *by themselves:* so long as they perceptibly continue to improve the disease state, even though improvement is gradual; for so long as the good effects continue with the indicated doses, the remedy must not be disturbed and stopped by any new remedy.[230] Kent advises: so long as curative action can be obtained, and even though the symptoms have changed, provided the patient is improving, hands off. Whenever in doubt, wait. It is a rule, after you have gone through a series of potencies, never to leave that remedy until one or more doses of a higher potency have been given and tested; but when that dose of a higher potency has been given and tested without effect...a change is necessary.[231]

Before deciding to administer a different remedy, the practitioner must be convinced beyond doubt that:

- The patient has settled firmly into a changed state of mental, emotional and physical suffering.
- The new symptoms experienced are permanent and not fleeting.
- The new picture of suffering is significantly different from the original characteristic symptom image totality upon which the first or previous prescription was based.
- The original treatment plan changes, e.g. the patient's ongoing longstanding suffering is interrupted by the onset of an acute, severe life-threatening upper-respiratory condition, or debilitating injury.

Only change the remedy if the symptoms have changed dramatically; but while the patient is improving, even though they may still experience some remaining original symptoms, do not interfere with the response of the vital force to that remedy; never ever change it. Leave the remedy and the vital force alone to expedite complete recovery.

If the patient reaches the end of a ascending potency scale but the remaining symptoms indicate the patient still needs the same remedy, do not desert that remedy. The vital force responded

---

[230] Dr. S. Hahnemann, *The Chronic Diseases: Their Peculiar Nature and Their Homœopathic Cure*

[231] Dr. J.T. Kent, *Lectures on Homœopathic Philosophy*

curatively to that potency scale. Therefore, it should not be changed. A reinvigorated more receptive vital force will respond well to reascending a potency scale.

Understanding when to change remedies is difficult. The heart is always in the mouth. To avoid changing remedies improperly, and inadvertently interrupt the curative effect of an earlier accurate prescription, follow these simple guidelines:

- In centesimal dosing, when there is improvement then the original symptoms return unchanged or diminished in frequency, duration and intensity, or one or more of the original symptoms have disappeared, then the first remedy selection is correct.

- In LM/Q dosing, when the patient improves at the beginning of dosing, the first remedy selection is correct
- Never change a remedy in haste without careful consideration and a very clear and logical reason.

- Never change remedies to hasten cure. For clearest instructions about what to do, observe and be guided by the patient's vital force as it expresses itself through the appearance, disappearance and reappearance of symptoms

- Never change a remedy when the existing symptoms change only slightly

- Always prescribe on the symptom totality rather than on a single symptom

- If the life force energy responds curatively to a remedy, do not desert that remedy

- Never *ever* change the remedy while the patient improves

- Never change the remedy when the symptoms change only slightly

- Never prejudge a state of suffering or its outcome

- Never decide beforehand what the next remedy or dose might be without a thorough re-examination of the patient

- Never assume that because a particular sequence of remedies and doses worked well for one person in one state of suffering e.g. eczema, the same sequence will work in all similar states of (eczema) suffering

- Never change the remedy when the symptom picture is moving

- Never desert a remedy that has acted curatively until after the remedy that produced the curative response has been tried in several ascending potencies and there has been no improvement at all in any of the mental, emotional or physical spheres of the original symptom image totality, *and* striking new symptoms appear and form a clear permanent change from the original symptom image totality and the patient's suffering intensifies.

13

Best Practice Checklist

"The physician who is most successful is he who will first heal for the love of healing, who will practice first to verify his knowledge and perform his use for the love of it. I have never known such a one to fail. This love stimulates him to continue, not to be discouraged with his first failures, and leads him to success in simple things first, and then in greater things. If he did not have an unusual affection for it, he would not succeed in it. An artist once was asked how it was that he mixed his paints so wonderfully, and he replied, 'with brains, sir.' So one may have all the knowledge of Homœopathy that it is possible for a human being to have, and yet be a failure in applying that art in its beauty and loveliness. If he has no affection for it, it will be seen to be a mere matter of memory and superficial intelligence. As he learns to love it, and dwell upon it as the very life of him, then he understands it is an art and can apply it in the highest degree."[232]

To treat each patient judiciously and rationally consider these points carefully:

- Avoid carelessness, laziness and levity.[233]
- Quiet thought hones the intellect.

---

[232] Dr. J.T. Kent, *Lectures on Homœopathic Philosophy*

[233] Dr. S. Hahnemann, *The Chronic Diseases: Their Peculiar Nature and Their Homœopathic Cure*

- Always think and observe before making decisions and taking action
- Let the principles guide your thought process
- Refuse to act impulsively, compulsively, routinely, out of fear or because you are feeling under pressure
- No prescription can be made for any patient until careful and prolonged study of the case has been completed
- Always investigate and prescribe for the whole state of the patient rather than a part of the patient's state
- It is hazardous and dangerous to administer a medicine without knowing the individual's constitution—the underlying influence of inherent predispositions to illness
- Ensure the symptom totality is the only basis for each remedy and dose selection
- Ensure the potency scale, dose and intervals between doses, accurately reflects the remaining prevailing strength or weakness of the patient's vital force
- The interval between doses stands next in importance only to the selection of the right remedy.[234]
- In the homœopathic treatment of long-term illness with centesimal doses, it is a fundamental rule, to let the action of the remedy come to an undisturbed conclusion while improvement still perceptibly progresses, so long as it visibly advances cure. This method forbids any new prescription any interruption by another medicine and forbids the immediate repetition of the same remedy.[235]
- After prescribing more than one remedy without achieving a curative response, stop. Do not continue. Watch and wait patiently for the development of characteristic individualising symptoms

---

[234] Dr. H. Farrington, *Homœopathy and Homœopathic Prescribing*

[232] Dr. S. Hahnemann, *The Chronic Diseases: Their Peculiar Nature and Their Homœopathic Cure*

- Trust the vital force of nature to communicate its needs through the language of symptoms.
- Never prescribe more than one remedy at a time; to do so creates confusion and violates Hahnemann's single remedy rule; it will be impossible to know with certainty which remedy produced a curative or non-curative response, which remedy should be repeated and which should not be repeated. This muddies the waters when considering when, why or how to make the correct second and further prescriptions
- Never consider a homœopathic dose of medicine too small to affect the patient and produce a response
- Before each new dose of medicine is to be given, the practitioner must be convinced of its usefulness.[236]
- In LM/Q potency dosing, select a single uncombined remedy and begin dosing. Monitor patient frequently to assess progress and, according to the response of the vital force, promptly adjust the frequency and amount (teaspoon, coffee spoon) as necessary
- Never give the patient several doses of the medicine to take with him so that he may take them himself at certain intervals, without considering whether this repetition may be injurious.[237]
- Avoid hasty, premature prescriptions
- Avoid practising isopathy or allopathy instead of homœopathy
- Honesty is the best policy. Explain to the patient how and why each error occurred and how it will be rectified.

---

[236]Dr. S. Hahnemann, *The Chronic Diseases: Their Peculiar Nature and Their Homœopathic Cure*

[237] Ibid.

Bibliography

Samuel Hahnemann MD

The *Materia Medica Pura*, 1811–1821 Arnold, Dresden.

The Organon of Medicine, Sixth Edition, 1922, Boericke Tafel.

The Chronic Diseases: Their Peculiar Nature Their Homœopathic Cure, 1828–1830, Arnold, Dresden.

Lesser Writings of Samuel Hahnemann, Edited by Robert Ellis Dudgeon, MD, 1852 William Radde.

James Tyler Kent MD

Lectures on Homœopathic Philosophy, 1900, Examiner Printing House, Lancaster, PA.

A Repertory of Homœopathic Materia Medica, 1897–1899, Examiner Printing House, Lancaster, PA.

Miscellaneous

A Compend of the Principles of Homœopathy. William Boericke, MD, 1896, Boericke Runyon.

The Genius of Homœopathy, Stuart N. Close, MD 1924, Boericke Tafel.

The Therapeutic Pocket Book. C. Von Boenninghausen, 1846.

Homœopathy and Homœopathic Prescribing, Harvey Farrington, MD, 1955.

The Principles and Art of Cure by Homœopathy, Herbert A. Roberts, MD, 1936 Homœopathic Publishing Company.

Kent's New Remedies, Clinical Cases, Lesser Writings, Aphorisms, and Precepts, Compiled by W. W. Sherwood, MD 1926, Erhart Karl

ABOUT THE AUTHOR

Born in England, Nicola Henriques began researching homœopathy in the early 1980s and received her Licentiate degree with honours, from the London College of Classical Homœopathy in 1993. Prior to that she was a journalist. Nicola practises Dr. Samuel Hahnemann's original medical system of homœopathy devoid of divergence and stripped of embellishments. She maintains a select clinical practice and offers occasional private continuing practitioner development tutorials. The author's other non-fiction books include *Women on Menopause: A Practical Guide to a Positive Transition; Crossroads to Cure: The Homeopath's Guide to Second Prescription; Release The Vital Force: The Exact Science and Art of Homœopathic Patient Examination.*

For more information visit:
www.nicolahenriques.com